OUR KIND
of
PEOPLE

———◁○▷———

Thoughts on the HIV/AIDS
Epidemic

Uzodinma Iweala

JOHN MURRAY

First published in Great Britain in 2012 by John Murray (Publishers)
An Hachette UK Company

1

© Uzodinma Iweala 2012

Where necessary, names and locations have been changed
to protect the privacy of people interviewed.

Designed by William Ruoto

A CIP catalogue record for this title is available from the British Library

ISBN 978-0-71952-340-3
TPB ISBN 978-0-71952-350-2
Ebook ISBN 978-1-84854-519-9

Printed and bound by Clays Ltd, St Ives plc

John Murray policy is to use papers that are natural, renewable
and recyclable products and made from wood grown in sustainable forests.
The logging and manufacturing processes are expected to conform to
the environmental regulations of the country of origin.

John Murray (Publishers)
338 Euston Road
London NW1 3BH

www.johnmurray.co.uk

FOR THOSE WHO HAVE LIVED

*Dalle quali cose e da assai altre a queste simiglianti o mag-
giori nacquero diverse paure e imaginazioni in quegli che
rimanevano vivi, e tutti quasi a un fine tiravano assai
crudele, ciò era di schifare e di fuggire gl'infermi e le lor
cose; e così faccendo, si credeva ciascuno a sé medesimo salute
acquistare.*

In which circumstances, not to speak of many others
of a similar or even graver complexion, divers appre-
hensions and imaginations were engendered in the
minds of such as were left alive, inclining almost all
of them to the same harsh resolution, to wit, to shun
and abhor all contact with the sick and all that belonged to them, thinking thereby to make each his
own health secure.

> —GIOVANNI BOCCACCIO, *The Decameron*,
> TRANS. J. M. RIGG

Stop AIDS. Fight AIDS.

> —FEMI KUTI

CONTENTS

JEROME

You know this story:

They called him Jerome. At least, he was popularly known as Jerome. I get the feeling that he was one of those people whom everyone knows but no one knows much about, including his real name— one of those guys who are so public that for the world they cease to have a private, inner life. There he was at the beer parlor, drink in hand, some girl giving him her undivided attention. There he was at the weddings he loved to crash, his hair barbed Cameroon style—what they might call a flattop in the United States—dressed "corporate," as they called it in those days, in a fitted suit, armpits patchy with sweat from the heat, and a freshly pressed dress shirt complete with a broad tie that hung from his neck to just above his shiny belt buckle. To Nigerians, the Cameroonians knew style, knew how to party, knew their way around women. Jerome wasn't Cameroonian, but maybe he should have been: he came from Cross River State in southern Nigeria, which shares a border with Cameroon.

He worked in construction—doing what, I'm

not sure anyone really knows. Like so many others, he came to Abuja when the city was still in its embryonic stages, more grassland and scrub brush than roads, houses, and government buildings. The earliest arrivals came by force. They were civil servants serving at the pleasure of a president, a military dictator who, after surviving a coup attempt in the crowded, congested, and unforgiving port city of Lagos, had accelerated plans to move the capital to a brand-new location in the dead center of Nigeria. They came because their jobs—indeed, the smooth functioning of the nation—depended on it. Others, like Jerome, came by choice. A new city was rising from the fields. There were jobs. There was money, real money to be made.

And money to be spent. Abuja was bush: not too much around for families to do, so the families stayed at home in their various states while the men, rich and poor, spent their money at brukutu joints, drinking the strong, freshly brewed Guinea corn (sorghum) liquor that gave the establishments their names. They sat on benches beneath the thatched roofs of open-air gazebos built in impromptu clusters, watching one another stagger around, their chatter growing louder and louder with the force of their drink. Away from their families, they would go to prostitutes. Jerome liked prostitutes—the thrill, the release of tension. He would take his friends, some of them much younger than he, to the back alleys and narrow passages between rattan and sackcloth huts where rainwater mixed with wastewater from the washing, where women, young and not so young, in tight spandex shirts that accentuated their cleavage, in leggings or jeans that emphasized their behinds, stood waiting for all manner of men and their money.

Jerome always had money, definitely enough for himself. Usually he had enough to help a friend inside those dimly lit rooms with their single mattresses and brightly colored plastic buckets for the necessary postcoital ablutions.

"Have fun!" he would encourage them. And he would have fun. "Work hard, play harder," the saying goes. That was Jerome. He worked. He played and he played.

Nobody saw it coming, least of all Jerome.

Her name was Agatha. She was young, probably not more than sixteen years old, but pretty in an adult way. Her body was developed beyond her years, and yet she still had a freshness that older women who looked like her had long since lost. She appeared one day in Jerome's compound at an apartment not far from his. She, like many other young village girls, probably had been sent up from her village down south by her parents to live with an uncle and his wife, to do house chores for them, and to care for their kids. In return, she would receive training, hopefully further her education, and at some point begin contributing to the upkeep of the parents who'd brought her into this world, helping them to support her siblings, who would also need to better themselves away from the backwater of Cross River State.

Who knows what first happened between them, whether it was a glance or a smile, or maybe one overheard the other speaking in their native southern tongue—a refreshing sound in Abuja, full of northern Hausa speakers—and intrigued, struck up a conversation. Everyone who knew them knows that things progressed quickly. She didn't really stand a chance, a naive village girl away from home, up against a suave, maybe even slick, city guy who had known many women. Like Diego Maradona, the Argentine soccer star, he dribbled her this way and that, they said, inviting her over to eat food that he—a grown man!—had cooked. He'd give her money, small amounts that didn't add up to anything but that to a young village girl seemed enormous. He would tell her to ask him for anything she needed as they sat waiting for the night to fall over the city. And Jerome would make love to the girl. He would play rough with her. Then he would fill her head with "sweet talks": "Agatha. You will be my future wife."

As they say in Nigeria, she now knew man.

Agatha's uncle noticed the change: disregard for the household chores, haughtiness when responding to simple questions, a sloppiness creeping into her work. He knew there was something. He had already caught her at Jerome's house twice earlier when she should have been at home working. Fearing that the girl would run off or get pregnant, her uncle promptly gathered her belongings and sent her south, back to the village, so that if she got pregnant, her father could not say it happened on his watch.

Maybe it was Jerome who didn't stand a chance against this fresh-faced and ever-so-gentle girl who no doubt reminded him of home, who had stilled something inside him, tamed the party animal, even if only for a moment. His friends thought that she had planted in him thoughts of the future and a desire to be responsible, because his behavior changed. He waited after she left. Maybe he even went back to his old ways, but it wasn't the same. As soon as he collected his monthly salary from the construction company, he traveled home to Cross River and then to Agatha's village, where he told her father that he wanted to marry her and bring her to Abuja.

Jerome would later tell his friends that the conversation was almost surreal. He stood there with the old man and stated his intentions—never mind that the girl was still young—as Agatha watched.

Then Agatha's father turned to her and asked, "Do you know this man?"

"Yes. I know him," she said softly but confidently.

"Did he discuss with you, say he want marry you?"

"He tell am before. Him say if these people should return me home, he will come bring me back to Abuja."

"Do you like to marry him?"

"Yes!"

"Then go."

It was unlikely that Agatha's father would object. For people in the village, Abuja meant money, and the way Jerome looked—the hair, the suit, the shoes—who wouldn't send his daughter away with him?

Jerome took Agatha back to Abuja, and not long after that, she got pregnant and had a baby girl. Very soon after, she became pregnant again and delivered a baby boy. That's when the problems started.

Agatha fell ill, but Jerome didn't want anybody to know. He hid Agatha, stopped her from attending the women's association meetings that the Cross River indigenes in Abuja had set up. He refused to take her to the hospital. His closest friends didn't understand why. Did he not have money for the hospital? Was he ashamed? Was something else going on in that house? But people noticed Agatha's absence. A couple of friends came round to check on her and found the poor girl suffering, unable to nurse her baby boy because one of her breasts had swollen tremendously. It continuously leaked pus—enough to fill a good-size saucer. Still Jerome refused to send the girl to the hospital until finally the breast burst open, leaving him no choice. He took her to the hospital, where they cleaned the wound, but he was unable to care for her and the two children and also continue to work. So he sent them home, back to her village, where her family could look after her, nurse her back to health.

Despite treatment at the hospital, she didn't get better. And the new baby, Jerome's first son, also seemed sick, weak, unable to grow. The boy soon died. Agatha grew weaker. Then she, too, died.

Jerome didn't know when Agatha died. His friends had to tell him one night in Mararaba, an Abuja suburb. They called him to come. It was late and the air was full of the scent of brewing brukutu, humming with conversation and the sounds of the roaming Hausa bards who beat, plucked, and sang out songs of praise and tales of sadness on their one- or two-string harps and small goatskin drums. No one wanted to say it. They sat quietly with Jerome, taking in how this vibrant man had, in recent months, become a shadow of himself physically. What was bothering him? they wondered. Was it stress? Was it Agatha's sickness? They were worried that he wouldn't accept the news, or worse still, that he wouldn't be able to take the news. He looked so weak. But you can only sweat silently for so long.

"You're a man," they told him as they sat with their brukutu. "There's nothing to hide from you. Your wife has passed."

Something wasn't right with Jerome, and it wasn't just the news that his wife had died. Of course, that would change any man. But Jerome's condition was something more than grief. It wasn't odd that he hadn't been out to drink or party in some time. His friends assumed he was mourning his wife. But he had even stopped going to work. He stayed at home alone. Those who knew him well saw the changes the most. There was Jerome, emaciated, with sunken eyes and skin that seemed to relinquish yet another shade of brown with each day. Every time he wanted to pass gas, he soiled himself. He didn't want to be seen in public—him, Jerome, a whole Jerome reduced and continuously reducing.

They begged him to go to the hospital; they begged him to submit himself for blood tests so doctors might determine the cause—beyond the bad luck of losing his wife and child. At Asokoro General Hospital, a collection of low-lying buildings in the center of the city, they drew his blood and admitted him to the wards.

The doctor was a young man. He entered the room with a worried look and drew in a long, slow breath. "Who is this person Jerome?" the doctor asked.

One of them answered, "It is my brother, my good friend, from the same side."

The doctor spoke again, and slowly. "Wow. OK. There is nothing to hide from you. Before, we hide it. Now we don't hide anything. Your friend has a bad deadly disease and he allowed it to go far, to destroy many things in his body. He has this new reigning disease HIV and AIDS. It is now gone far, to the extent that the blood system is now weak. So there is nothing we can do. If you keep moving him from hospital to hospital, it's just a waste of funds."

So Jerome's friends did the only thing they could do. They took him back to Cross River, to his village. That's where he gave up. That's how Jerome passed on.

His baby boy was gone. His wife was gone. He

too was now gone. And somewhere out there, his daughter is left behind to grow up without parents.

You know this story. You have heard it many times before. This is the story of HIV/AIDS in Africa.

Or is it?

For the rest of the world, Africa's story has been one of exploitation, famine, floods, war, and now tragic demise as a result of HIV/AIDS. This troubles me. Despite growing up with exposure to both the Western world and Africa—in particular, Nigeria, where my family is from—even I sometimes succumb to thinking of Africa as a place beyond hope and Africans as sad creatures destined to slow-dance with adversity. I should know better, because I have experienced the continent, at least my small corner of it, as a place characterized by something other than tragedy, but it is hard not to think negatively, especially when the vast majority of media from the past few hundred years—the explorers' accounts, novels, newspaper articles, documentaries—have focused on Africa's pain. Though a relatively new disease, HIV/AIDS and its stories have again brought to the foreground a whole set of images and stereotypes about Africans, our societies, our bodies, our sexualities.

Many of these representations of Africa are deployed to elicit sympathy and encourage assistance with HIV/AIDS and other issues. Often, however, they unknowingly encourage the opposite, distancing and disconnection, because they provide an image of Africa and Africans to which few people can relate. The lives and voices of real people, who like everybody else in this world find ways to cope with adversity, are often lost amid the drumbeat of deprivation and demise. This confuses me. At times, this angers me. While I understand that Africa—its countries, its people—has endured a fair amount of adversity, the tragic Africa is not the only continent I know.

I grew up in Washington, DC, but my family is from Nigeria. From the moment I was born, each summer my parents would take my three siblings and me "home" to visit family. These trips were an often confusing exposure to the dynamic milieu of personalities, cultures, and languages, the stark contrast of privilege and poverty, and the innovation that such a mixture encourages. The Africa I got to know through summers spent in Nigeria while growing up was one of both struggle and promise. It was a place where issues like HIV/AIDS were part of a complex existence. I don't want to minimize the scope and impact of the epidemic, just to say that it's not all we are.

In early 2006, a year and a half after I graduated from college, I began working on health policy issues in sub-Saharan Africa with the Millennium Villages Project, a comprehensive development program headquartered at Columbia University and the United Nations with the mission of alleviating poverty and associated ills in sub-Saharan Africa. I was a very junior employee, mostly acting as an assistant to the team coordinating the project's health programs. I was exposed to many aspects of health care in Africa, the different diseases, the lack of adequate health systems, and the language used to describe conditions on the continent. At the headquarters in New York, however committed we were to presenting a different view of Africa to the world, the rhetoric would sometimes slide into the usual images of helpless Africans and their saviors from abroad. When I spent time with our local experts in the field, I often found myself in an awkward position. They would complain bitterly to me about those people in New York who didn't really respect Africans. "Those white people," one of my colleagues said to me, "they really don't think very highly of us at all." His words seem harsh, but perhaps I can explain why he might arrive at this conclusion.

In the spring of 2006, in New York, I attended a talk about HIV/AIDS sponsored by the Earth Institute at Columbia University. The speaker stepped to a podium in the cavernous Lerner Auditorium bathed in bright white stage lights. His voice tremulous with concern and amplified by large speakers, he painted such a dire picture of HIV/AIDS in Africa that it seemed only a matter of months before all 800 million sub-Saharan Africans would contract the virus and perish.

"People don't have access to information. People don't have access to medication," I remember him thundering as the mostly white, mostly Western audience sighed in sorrowful agreement. "People are dropping like flies."

I sat up. I remember scribbling those words on a program that I have long since lost.

"Dropping like flies" is an often used and, as a result, rather innocuous simile, but in that context it made me wonder: is this how Africans are considered, as insects, animals, not human? Is resorting to a metaphor of inhumanity the only way to register the magnitude of the problem unfolding on such a vast scale before us? In fairness, "dropping like flies" can be used to describe any set of people, but historical associations of Africans with animals make such language very complicated. Sometimes it can even be perceived as outright disrespectful.

On the other hand, what does it mean to say that

33.4 million people in the world are HIV positive and 28.2 million of those in sub-Saharan Africa? What does it mean to say that 1.8 million people in Africa died last year as a result of the virus and its effects? There is no love or loss in a decimal point, no resilience and no redemption. Statistics, however beautifully rendered in tables or graphs or charts, cannot even begin to relay the tragedies and triumphs of this situation. Such large numbers defy comprehension and flout nuance, leaving people to seek explanation in simple narratives that stand as symbols for the epidemic:

> There was a man from the country who went to work in the city. He slept with a prostitute and contracted HIV. When he returned home, he slept with his wife. Then she died. Then he died. Now their children are orphans.

Tragedy occurs without bounds and death piles upon death. Numbers feature prominently while the characters remain faceless. These stories exist, but they are not the only stories Africa has to tell about its experience with HIV/AIDS.

It would be too easy to write a polemic against past and even present depictions of Africans and our relationship to HIV and AIDS. There are too many instances in which egregiously racist beliefs and subtle prejudices have colored both descriptions of Africa's HIV/AIDS epidemic and the responses to it. There are too many examples of how sensationalism—even when well-meaning—has impeded our understanding of this disease and the people it affects, creating distance where none need exist, making a terrible fantasy of something very real.

As I sat in that auditorium surrounded by a sea of well-meaning white Western colleagues and luminaries in the field of international health swooning in the presence of this powerful speaker, I suddenly felt very aware of and protective of my African-ness. I began to wonder if there was a way to consider the hard truths of the HIV/AIDS epidemic in Africa and to impress upon people the urgent need for action in a way that was fundamentally humanizing and empowering for those living in the epicenter of this crisis. I thought I might be able to develop a better understanding of what HIV/AIDS means and how we can deal with it by spending time in Nigeria, in a country that is home to one fifth of sub-Saharan Africa's population and the third-largest population of HIV-positive people in the world. I hoped that this would give me an indication of the epidemic's impact on the whole region. I thought I could find answers to my questions in a few months, but my exploration turned into a four-year journey, with multiple trips between Nigeria and the United States, that has changed my understanding of the HIV virus, its epidemic, and the real people it affects. I had no idea what I was about to discover.

AIDS IS REAL

A IDS is real," the driver said, pondering the no-tion for a moment while gnawing the end of a bleached wood chewing stick. He spat a gob of wet pulp out the car window before turning back to me. He was probably the driver for one madam living in the same Victoria Garden City neighborhood of La-gos where my family has a house. Now that he had dropped his employer at work, he had the time for a leisurely kindness otherwise unknown to constantly grinding Lagosians. I had never met him before, and I probably shouldn't have accepted. In Lagos you don't get into just anybody's car. All the same, I was appreciative when he offered me a ride after seeing me walking from our house to the Lekki Expressway where I could catch a taxi. I fidgeted in the passenger seat of the air-conditioned SUV.

In the distance, the mini-skyscrapers of Victoria Island and down at the city center near the marina shimmered against an embankment of low clouds, and I remembered an uncle's sarcastic statement that from afar, Lagos actually looks like a wonderful city. Like New York, Lagos is a city of islands. From the air, you can see the massive lagoon that separates the sections of the city on the mainland from the two large islands in the Atlantic Ocean, and the city's latticework of paved highways, occasional red-earth side streets, and tin roofs looks deceptively peaceful. In truth, this megalopolis, though impressive in scale, is frustrating beyond belief; it simmered around us as we sat in the famous Lagos go-slow (traffic jam). Cars and trucks stretched for miles ahead of us toward the city center and miles behind us toward its outskirts, where developers couldn't build houses fast enough for an exponentially growing population. Street hawkers roamed among idling vehicles and thrust everything from chilled soft drinks in perspiring bottles to steering wheel covers up against car windows. Lagos, the joke goes, is the one city in the world where, because of the traffic, you can accomplish all of your shopping on the way to the market. That morning the only forward movement came from the *okadas* (motorbike taxis), which buzzed through tight spaces between cars, leaving behind a trail of suffocating black exhaust as they passed.

I was on my way to see Rolake Odetoyinbo, the head of Positive Action for Treatment Access (PATA), an advocacy group for causes related to HIV/AIDS. I was going to be late, even by Nigerian standards. PATA's offices were in the Ikeja section of Lagos on the mainland. Though I had budgeted two hours for what should be a half-hour drive, an accident on the road blocked movement. As the car idled in traffic, the driver and I had struck up a conversation about HIV/AIDS.

"AIDS is real," he said again after he removed the chewing stick from his mouth. His eyes flashed with a knowing excitement before he spoke again. "It has been here for generations with our forefathers," he said in the blasé tone of someone for whom besiegement is ordinary. "We have a word for it. *Atogbe*," he mouthed the Yoruba word slowly.

"*Atogbe*," I repeated and then wrote it down. He sighed appreciatively.

"Yes. *Atogbe*, someone who urinate until he die. And until when the death comes, he has six or seven sickness at the same time. We have known this thing since the olden days, but now the whites, them come call it AIDS."

The first reported case of AIDS in Nigeria was diagnosed in 1985 and presented at the second International AIDS Conference in Paris the following year. According to the case reports, the patient in question was a thirteen-year-old female street hawker from Lagos. I could find out little about this girl or how she contracted the virus that causes AIDS—which at that time was called HTLV-III (human T-lymphotrophic virus III) or LAV (lymphadenopathy-associated virus), depending on whether you followed the American or the French researchers. I could determine only that it was in Lagos that HIV supposedly first appeared in Nigeria and, as far as some are concerned, from this city that HIV spread to the rest of the country.

"It is from those in the coasts, the towns like Lagos, Port Harcourt. Big cities with the white men, the seamen, those who work with the ships, or soldiers—police, too," an old retired civil servant said to me as we sat on his veranda sipping bottles of Coke. We had met in a small town in eastern Nigeria. "At first, when this thing was noted in this country, our people, they discountenanced it. They said, 'What is that? What is AID? Oh! Nah—sickness for the whites and those up there.' Some, in order to enjoy themselves how they want, they say there is nothing like AIDS."

When it first appeared in Nigeria, AIDS was rejected as a nonissue by the successive military governments, as well as by the general public. At less than ten thousand dollars, the original budget for the first AIDS-related government body in Nigeria, the National Expert Advisory Committee on AIDS (NEACA), was laughable. The military dictators took a stance similar to that of other African leaders at the time: AIDS is not a problem here. In popular thought up until the late 1990s, AIDS was also considered a nonissue, sometimes referred to as the American Invention to Discourage Sex, if referred to at all.

It wasn't until the late 1990s that Nigeria—indeed, most of Africa—began to wake up to the crisis brewing in our midst. I remember the summer of 1997, when the great Afro-beat musician Fela Kuti died and over a million people marched his coffin down the streets of Lagos. I was fifteen then and remember watching the procession on television with my family in my uncle's living room. There was total silence. "Fela," said Olikoye Ransome-Kuti, his brother and the former minister of health, "had died of AIDS." People couldn't believe it. For weeks afterward, there were whispers: "How can a great man like Fela die of AIDS? It's not possible!"

But the revelation that Fela had lived with and ultimately died from HIV/AIDS did spark some change. Also important was Nigeria's return to democracy and the election of Olusegun Obasanjo, who was very concerned about HIV/AIDS as president. I remember when billboards with public service announcements about it (now ubiquitous throughout the country) first appeared on buildings and by highways. They displayed slogans like AIDS NO DEY SHOW FOR FACE next to the smiling face of musician

Femi Kuti, Fela's famous son, or KNOW YOUR STATUS next to images of happy couples in traditional dress. Newly elected President Obasanjo spoke openly of the "HIV/AIDS pandemic that continues to bring havoc, misery and hopelessness on humanity, especially in Africa where the pandemic is threatening to wipe out entire generations." He made public appeals to the citizens and members of the military and police to get tested. Something, however small, in the country's attitude toward HIV/AIDS was changing.

I could hear it in the discussions about HIV on the radio or in the comments my cousins in college made about safe sex. Once, during a visit home the summer after I graduated from college, I overheard two gentlemen pondering the process of HIV transmission in a Lagos nightclub: "If a man get am and a woman get am, then any child they get must surely catch am." His companion offered a laughing rebuke. "No. No. No. It neva pass like that."

By the early part of this century, HIV/AIDS had become part of the national consciousness. Certainly I could see now, as this kind driver and I rolled slowly along the main thoroughfares of a hustling, bustling, choked, and congested city, it had become part of the landscape as well. Billboards and posters lined the highway. I saw the universal awareness symbol, a red ribbon, painted boldly on the backs of transport trucks. AIDS was now real to Nigerians but, as it is to most of the world, in an abstract, "I've heard about it and know it's there" kind of way.

The demographics of the HIV/AIDS epidemic in Nigeria and worldwide are such that people need not knowingly encounter someone who is HIV positive every day. The most recent data collected by the Nigerian Ministry of Health reveal that about 4 percent of Nigeria's population is HIV positive. This is a small percentage when compared to the 20 percent of the population that is positive in countries like Botswana or South Africa. However, 4 percent of Nigeria's 150 million people means approximately 3 million Nigerians are living with HIV, the third-largest population of positive people in the world. With such enormous numbers, it seems inconceivable that someone could not know an HIV-positive person, but Nigeria is a geographically and demographically large country. Likewise, though there are approximately 34 million positive people in the world, this is actually less than half of 1 percent of the total global population. This means that most people in the world today have not and will not knowingly encounter someone living with HIV. Under such circumstances, it is hard to convey the diversity of experiences that constitute the reality of HIV. In my own case, when I started writing this book, despite having a background in health and time spent working on the HIV/AIDS epidemic in Africa, I was not close to anyone of known positive status. I had yet to see what the day-to-day reality of HIV/AIDS in Nigeria was like.

One of the first conversations I had about HIV/AIDS in Nigeria when I first started writing was with my good friend Femi Adegoke. At the time, he had just finished a master's degree in public health at Harvard and returned to Abuja to work for Columbia University's International Center for AIDS Care and Treatment Programs. He has since moved on to work for a number of HIV/AIDS-focused organizations in Nigeria. Indirectly, he was the reason I ended up getting an appointment with Rolake Odetoyinbo. One night in early 2007 as we sat on the rooftop bar of the British Council, a common hangout for diplomats, expats, and aid workers in Abuja, watching the power flicker across different neighborhoods in the common practice of load sharing, he said to me that in Nigeria, "We don't see AIDS patients. We need to be faced with this reality to move forward. We need to see these things every day."

That same week, there happened to be a very visible HIV/AIDS presence in the capital. Every two years, the major groups involved in HIV/AIDS-related work convene at a conference sponsored by the National Agency for the Control of AIDS (NACA), the government body charged with rationalizing and coordinating Nigeria's response to the epidemic. With community-based organizations, advocacy groups, NGOs, and state government agencies traveling to Abuja from each of Nigeria's thirty-six states, as well as a strong representation from international organizations, the conference is anything but a regular affair. It is not designed to represent the daily reality of HIV/AIDS, but to allow those who work on the Nigerian epidemic the chance to come together to share experiences, debate related issues, and ultimately speak with one voice about the direction the country needs to take to improve the lives of people living with HIV/AIDS and prevent more infections from occurring. Femi urged me to attend, saying this would be the best place to gain a broad understanding of HIV in Nigeria and perhaps meet people who might be of good help.

Later that week, I drove to the Abuja International Conference Centre, where the meetings were already under way. I had been to the massive structure, with its sweeping arc of a roof and immaculate glass facade, a couple of years earlier for the wedding reception of a cousin. Then, the speckled red granite floor of the grand entrance hall had boasted a red carpet and numerous tables covered in white cloths and pink napkins. Bridesmaids in pink danced among the tables, inviting all who were seated to join in the festivities and move to loud music echoing from the wall speakers.

The day of the conference was an altogether more serious affair. The entrance hall still sparkled but remained unfurnished. Instead it bustled with people in dark suits or traditional Nigerian prints, attaché cases or files of documents in hand or under arm. The attendees were mostly domestic. They stood in clusters, locked in serious conversations. They folded their arms across their chests or cupped their chins in the space between thumb and index finger. Occasionally greetings would break up the exchanges as smiles and laughter erupted when people working on similar issues in different parts of the country made their annual reconnections and collided into hugs and handshakes.

Femi had told me about the conference after the completion of registration, so I attended without accreditation. I slunk around the conference hall from table to table, picking up literature, pocketing brochures, and engaging in casual conversation with the representatives of various NGOs and SACAs (state AIDS control agencies) who had arranged their tables and booths to emphasize the strengths or needs of their various organizations. All of Nigeria's thirty-six states were represented. At the Kogi State table, tended by a wiry man with tinted lenses in his metal frames, the emphasis was on counseling and testing programs for sex workers. Kogi borders Abuja, and its capital, Lo-koja, sits near the confluence of the Niger and Benue Rivers. Any truck heading toward the southwest must pass through this city. Where there are long-haul truck drivers, the conventional wisdom goes, there are sex workers, and in these places, there tends to be a higher rate of HIV transmission. The Plateau State booth boasted a whole set of educational materials for primary schools, with a group of young women hardly enthusiastic to explain the process of creating them. They told me they were members of the National Youth Service Corps, recent university graduates completing a mandatory year of national service. Mass communication, not HIV/AIDS, was their specialty. They looked more disoriented than I was.

After an hour of wandering from table to table, I stumbled from the main hall back into the lobby with an armful of brochures and a pocketful of business cards. I had met a few interesting people, some of whom I intended to contact immediately, but for the most part, I was tired and confused. I recognized that there was a certain absurdity about not wanting to sensationalize the HIV/AIDS epidemic while desperately searching for some charismatic HIV-positive figure to introduce me to its reality. I had no idea where to begin. This overload of voices, colored brochures, screaming posters, and videos was not helping.

I made my way toward a set of stairs that led to an over-air-conditioned cafeteria. As I ascended, I briefly locked eyes with a young man with uncombed curls of hair, dressed in a dashiki and descending the staircase.

"Do I know you?" he asked.

"I don't think so," I stammered, concerned that he was a conference organizer who would realize that I had no right to be around and promptly usher me out.

"Dapo," he introduced himself, extending a hand. "I work with PATA." He noticed my blank look and added, "Positive Action for Treatment Access. We're based in Lagos. Who are you with?"

"Oh, I'm not really with anyone. Just trying to get an idea of what AIDS is really like in this country."

He nodded knowingly. "So you're a journalist."

I didn't answer. I didn't necessarily want this to be a journalistic endeavor, but journalist seemed more acceptable than "personal crusader" or "interested party."

"Well, I work for my sister Rolake, who founded the NGO. If your work brings you to Lagos, be in touch."

I had heard about Rolake Odetoyinbo but not her organization. She is a well-known and well-regarded

Nigerian AIDS activist who has had no qualms discussing her HIV-positive status on television, radio, and in the regular columns she writes for newspapers and magazines. I was in luck.

The PATA offices were in a dingy four-story building set back from the noise of Awolowo Way, a busy street in the Ikeja section of Lagos. The noise of the building's standby generator was relative calm compared to the horns of the traffic-clogged road yards away. It looked sturdy, but the structure had clearly seen better days, a condition that became all the more apparent when I entered a dimly lit staircase with plaster flaking off the walls. But inside the office, the sunlit rooms were a whirl of bright fabrics as women participating in a PATA-run support-group meeting flitted about with plates of food, conversing and laughing loudly over the unrelenting rumble of the generator two stories below. The walls were sparsely decorated with informational posters advertising new HIV medications and encouraging safe sex. Powerful standing fans made the posters flutter against the walls.

Rolake appeared moderately peeved, if also understanding of my tardiness.

"Go-slow," I muttered, invoking the traffic jam as an apology.

She offered me a plate from a table full of rice, fish and beef stews, and fried plantains. Then she led me to a corner of the room away from the commotion.

She was, as she had been described to me by a university student who had seen her speak in a seminar, "Big. Healthy-looking. An average person." Her round face was indeed full and healthy with smooth, plump cheeks that folded into creases under her eyes. She traveled constantly, and though she wore it well, the fatigue was still written on her face. Before she became an HIV/AIDS activist, Rolake was a relatively successful baker who sold her pastries in fast-food joints and other venues. It wasn't her ideal job—she had studied dramatic arts at one of Nigeria's premier universities—but her husband's career moved him from place to place, and she needed something flexible to earn money. She lived what she calls a relatively normal life until testing positive for HIV in 1998.

In an interview for the Nigerian newspaper *Punch*, she called the first four years after she tested positive the "worst years of my life" because "for four years I was waiting for death." She said, "I was so sure AIDS was going to kill me," and told the interviewer, "It was four years of living in fear, silence and stigma, not knowing what to do and not having access to the right information." Then in 2002, she attended an AIDS conference in Barcelona, and it changed her life. "I didn't know much about HIV. In fact, I wasn't open about my status. I went to Barcelona with the knowledge that HIV was a death sentence. I felt that while I was alive, let me just get the best out of life," she said in a 2004 interview with the Nigerian newspaper *Vanguard*. "The conference for me wasn't so exciting. It was the people I met that made the world of difference. I met people who had lived with HIV for 20 years and couldn't tell they had HIV. So Barcelona challenged my mentality. It also helped me see HIV/AIDS in a different light." In the *Punch* interview, she had said, "I realised that if I wanted to die, I could do a better job jumping in front of a moving train because HIV wasn't in a hurry to kill me."

Two months after she returned from Barcelona, tired of the silence, shame, and fear and wanting more from life, she gave an interview to a major newspaper disclosing her HIV status. Her life changed dramatically. From speaking to conferences and support groups, she went on to found PATA (Positive Action for Treatment Access), a group that seeks to empower women living with HIV and AIDS, prevent the transmission of HIV from mother to child, and build awareness and understanding of the epidemic in the general population.

"My face is the face of HIV," Rolake said to me as we struggled to get comfortable in metal folding chairs we had removed from a circle set up for the support-group meeting that was to follow. In many ways, she *is* a prominent internationally known face of HIV. She sits on a board at the powerful Global Fund to Fight AIDS, Tuberculosis and Malaria. She is a regular speaker at conferences around the world.

Her words brought to mind a poster produced by the Keep a Child Alive Campaign. The poster features a dozen American celebrities in face paint designed to simulate "African tribal markings," all set above the legends I AM AFRICAN in bright yellow and HELP US STOP THE DYING in danger red. It is one of the more offensive HIV ad campaigns I have encountered, something akin to a nouveau blackface that in one fell swoop manages to incorporate a whole host of stereotypes and negative ideas about the continent—the exoticization of the other and this idea of a primitive beauty, as well as the subtle, unintentional suggestion that to be African is to be HIV positive and thus close to the brink of death.

Rolake has consistently positioned herself against such messaging. "We"—Rolake opened her arms as she spoke to indicate the international activist community—"have sold ourselves short. We have created the impression that Africa is poor, hungry, beggarly children. And this glamorizing poverty to whip up sentiment and fund-raise? It's emotional blackmail. HIV is not a disease of the poor. It's a disease of the working class." I understood her words not as a denial of the link between HIV/AIDS and poverty but rather a statement that people with HIV/AIDS are not totally helpless creatures so far removed from life.

"My face won't bring money. But it should," she continued. "My face should tell you that if we have access to treatment, we will remain productive. That's what I want to do in my work, present a portrait of strength." It was hard not to be excited by her feistiness and aggressive pushback against the status quo, by her desire to reduce the representational distance between people who have HIV and people who do not.

"I don't want to go out and look like HIV," she told the *Vanguard* interviewer. "When we were hearing about AIDS 10 years ago, the picture was all gloom and doom. We were hearing of people dying in the UK and America. We don't hear that anymore. Is it that they've eradicated HIV/AIDS from that part of the world? No, they have access to treatment and HIV has stopped being a death sentence. It has become like high blood pressure, which has no cure but can be managed with medication. So for me, the most important issue is for HIV/AIDS to stop being a death sentence. We can live with HIV."

Rolake's work has gone a long way toward normalizing HIV/AIDS, for both those with positive status and the rest of the population, by presenting a reality that is not all sensation, gloom, hardship, and death. A recent university graduate I interviewed in Lagos told me that hearing her speak had transformed the way she thought about HIV/AIDS because people like to think that "people that die of AIDS or have HIV are dirty people, people that sleep around or do rubbish and stuff, not our kind of people," while Rolake just looked so normal. If her aim is to desensationalize the disease and therefore make it livable, tangible, and real for Nigerians and the world, then perhaps her relentless campaigning is generating results.

She stood up. My notebook hung open over one knee, pen secured safely in its binding. I had arrived too late for an extended discussion. She had her support group to attend to. Before she excused herself, she said, "If you want to know what things are really like, you should talk to women like these," and opened her palms toward the women assembling in their seats.

The reality of HIV/AIDS in Nigeria and Africa is a diversity of experiences. There is no archetypal story, no single defining theme. For all people who experience the disease, whether HIV positive or not,

the reality is influenced by who they are as individuals and the communities to which they belong. The
HIV/AIDS epidemic does not exist outside of regular life. Rather, it is shaped by regular life, just as it
shapes our everyday experiences.

A few months after I met Rolake, I visited a
woman named Hope who lived in the capital of Imo
State, a city called Owerri. Owerri is an eight-hour
road trip east of Lagos and sits in the middle of an area
of the country populated predominantly by members of my Igbo ethnic group. My father grew up in
a village only an hour away. When I was younger
and we used to do the grueling drive from Lagos
to my grandparents' village, Owerri was one of the
last stops along the way. It never seemed to come
fast enough. Whereas Lagos is all over-the-top grind
and hustle, with the larger-than-life atmosphere of a
developing world megalopolis, Owerri is much qui-
eter, "cooler," as people from the town like to say.
The city is definitely more laid-back. The buildings
don't rise as high. There are fewer car horns blasting
at any given moment, and all around there is green,
the remnants of what used to be massive primary-
growth rain forest.

Hope lived in a compound of several similarly
constructed one-story buildings in what appeared to
be an unfinished housing estate. These low houses

were partitioned into multiple one- or two-room living quarters with outdoor kitchens protected from the elements by low-hanging eaves. It seemed that work on the estate had halted some time ago, because rusting construction machinery, tractors, backhoes, and earthmovers sat disintegrating in pools of dark water. The grass that could grow shot up through bits of debris, a rich and lively green. Dragonflies buzzed around the waving grass stalks and above scattered puddles. Behind it all loomed the city's dilapidated cathedral.

Places like this are unsettling, but I was troubled more by my reaction to the surroundings than by the environment itself. This kind of place speaks of an unglamorous struggle where daily life is a steady stream of inconveniences—no running water, no electricity, and no money for a diesel generator, with the threat of catastrophe lurking in the background. As a person of relative privilege in Nigeria, I find such environments unsettling. They remind me of the extreme nature of my own privilege and how disconnected I am from the experiences of the many people in Nigeria who live on less than two dollars a day. At times I catch myself slipping into romanticizing the suffering, marveling at what seems an inhuman ability to survive what we call inhumane conditions. I struggled to collect my thoughts.

Hope saw me from her window and opened her door before I had a chance to knock. She had tried her best to make the hot, dark one-room apartment hospitable. Plastic flowers adorned the security bars guarding the window. Pictures in frames—her wedding day, children, and assorted other family—hung on shadowed walls. Still more stood atop a dusty television and sparkled when a little light touched them. She invited me to sit down on a purple couch striped by the light entering through the open window and cracked door. There was no electricity, thus no fan. A large hanging curtain that separated the area where she and her children slept from where we now sat languished in the stillness, shifting occasionally with a breath of air from outside.

"The time my husband was alive, we live in three-bedroom flat," she said almost as an apology. "We just use one room to pack foodstuffs. If you enter my house, you will just serve yourself—enjoy. You will see rice in bags, fruits, everything. Every week, he'll be giving me ten thousand naira and saying, 'Use it that anything you like you can buy.' My children, every three-three months, I will take them to market and get what they need. Weekend, I will take them to this fast-food joint, Mr. Bigg's. But now, there's nothing like that. I have to manage, as he's not around now."

I noticed for the first time just how young Hope looked. Her eyes were closed in remembrance. Her face was plain and without makeup. She wore her hair natural and unstyled, secured in a tight bun that stretched the skin of her forehead and emphasized her high cheekbones. She appeared to have weathered the stresses of life after her husband's death relatively well.

"Even as I'm here, I don't have anything doing. I'm just managing myself. The only thing I do now is to sell Pure Water around this place, NNPC [Nigerian National Petroleum Corporation] filling station. If I get something like three hundred naira or anything, I will just use it and manage. Then my parents do help me, but you know, even if they are giving you one million naira a day, you're supposed to have something doing."

She had settled now into a routine that included scraping together an income from her petty trading, raising two young teenagers, and focusing on her HIV treatments, all while living somewhat in the shadow of her previous life. Her apartment walls seemed to have an inordinate number of pictures from the past, mostly of her wedding. I soon found out why.

Hope sighed, reached for her wedding album beneath the glass coffee table, and carefully opened it before us. When she reached a picture of her and her husband standing on the red earth at the bottom of a staircase leading up to a double set of church doors, both of them dressed in a white that matched their broad bright smiles, she turned to me.

"He went for operation. There is one thing that do him on his head here. Look at it here," she said, pointing to a bulge atop her husband's cropped hair that transformed his otherwise round head into an oblong structure. "He wanted to remove it. In Nigeria here, before you do any operation—anything— any hospital that you enter, you must test that HIV test. They told us they would do test."

"This happened before your wedding?" I scrutinized her husband's face in the picture. "When did you get married?"

"I wedded in 2001—in a church."

"But," I said, looking at the two children, a boy and girl standing with her and her husband. They resembled the children in a photo hanging by a clock on the wall. "Your children . . ."

She stopped me with an anemic wave. "I did my traditional wedding 1993, and then I wedded in church in 2001 after getting my issue," she said and pointed to her children in the picture. "Here now, I'm up to twenty-something years before I wedded in church. I was fourteen when I did my traditional wedding."

Hope had grown up in a relatively strict household. Her father, a trader in the local markets, though loving, was perhaps driven to fear on behalf of his family as a result of his hyperacute sense of danger. Rather than have daughters subjected to the indignities of this world, namely premarital sex and all its risks, he decided that they would be better off married early—in Hope's case, very early.

"My dad, he do always say this is what he wants," she said. "He just put it in prayer, 'God, I don't want any of my daughter to stay here and become pregnant. My prayer is that if I train my children, let them grow up in a good way, that they may train me at the old age. It's better that they marry and go to their husband's place so that they will be more glad than to stay at home.'" This is not a typical sentiment among the Igbos, who tend to marry later in life. I could, however, understand the reasoning, the preference for an honorable marriage over the shame of a dishonorable pregnancy, or worse yet, a killer disease. His actions revealed desire for a solid definition of decency in a world of rapidly changing social and sexual mores.

Hope's older sister introduced her to the man who would become her husband. He was about fifteen years her senior and already established as a relatively successful tractor-trailer driver who shipped goods around for many of the important local politicians and businessmen.

"I don't know him before I went to his place," Hope made clear to me, meaning that she had not had sex with her husband. "I said, 'OK, you know that I'm still a small girl, quite all right, and you, you're older than me.' I asked him, 'Why did you decided to marry a small girl like this?' He say, it's how he decided. All those grown-up girls, he don't like the person that he will brought in. The person may not respect him. He will want to start from the smallest so that the small girl may respect him and he will teach that girl. It's just he wanted to brush the person up by hisself."

"You weren't afraid?" I asked.

"I was not afraid. How can I be afraid?"

She looked at me directly for the first time. Her eyes were clear and bright, even in the dimness, her face rough with something approaching indignation.

"No. I was not afraid, 'cause I go in to pray. After introduction, then he pay my bride price—just twenty thousand naira as of that 1993." She paused to emphasize the absurdity of inflation. In 1993 twenty thousand naira was almost a thousand dollars. Today the same sum is less than one hundred and fifty dollars.

"He now do my traditional wedding. Ah!" She rocked back and forth for a moment, her mind and body caught up in the music and celebration of so long ago. "They danced now! We called Band Eze. We invite them there. Another person, a singer, from Owerri—I do forget his name—we invite him too. It was very tough! I was happy! He pulled crowd. Even commissioners, they were there. The PDP [People's Democratic Party] chairman in this state, all of them are there."

She was smiling now and even clapped her hands when remembering the music they had played that day, almost fifteen years earlier. For a moment, I could see the woman she might have been before, excited, voluble, full of emotion that showed in her wide smile.

Hope's two children were born in quick succession after her marriage and life settled into a pattern of relative comfort and prosperity as her husband's business thrived, but it seemed that he was seldom around. Such are the lives of interstate truck drivers. Some years later, in 2001, probably after her husband had saved a good chunk of money, they decided to have what Nigerians call the white wedding. In Nigeria the traditional wedding is considered the most important ceremony. As my mother says, you can get married in as many churches as you want, but unless you have your traditional ceremony, no one will respect your union. If finances are tight, most people will do their traditional wedding first, and later, sometimes years later, when they find the money, they perform the white wedding.

"I wedded in January 2001. Then we discovered this thing September 2001," she explained. "At the moment they find that thing out, he was not happy. He said, 'Hai! What will I do?' I said, 'There's no problem. I'm your wife.' The moment he found out, the man, he got confused. If you're advising him, just relax, that the thing has never started—just relax—they just find it out, he said, 'No! A man like me, a popular person!' Because he do deal with big-big men. He say he won't stay watching himself let people know that he has this problem. It's better that he die. It's better he just die," she said softly. It was hard not to detect a hint of resentment in her appraisal of her late husband's behavior—as if his conduct was somehow unbecoming of a man of his status.

"Likewise, my own, I discover it by the year 2001, December. After they tested him, he said I should go, and I tested positive. When I discover it, I thought that my own has finished, but later, later on I could withstand it. First of all, I went to my pastor and say, 'Pastor! What is going on?' He say, 'Relax. Everything depends on God. With God, all things are possible,'" she said, again lost in those past moments, speaking quickly as if to get through the worst parts of a bad situation.

Their lives transformed from the usual work, children, and church to a new norm of seeking treatments and hiding their conditions. "Somebody directed me and my husband to Abuja," she said. "We went to a doctor there who promise is that he's going to do everything, that everything will be settled, that he can take care of that. We continue giving him money every time. Any trip—we were going there every month—we would go with one hundred and fifty thousand naira.* We started taking some root, something medicine. We take it over a year and there's no way, no improvement. Instead of improvement it would be going worst."

"Did your relationship with your husband change?" I asked. "Were you angry with him?"

"I wasn't harsh on him. I know that something may occur and let God give us a solution. No other thing. He was the one that worried himself, but I was not angry with him. I know that he didn't do me anything wrong.

"I used to advise him that he should take everything easy. He was thinking, thinking. Later-later,

---

* About one thousand dollars.

he just developed high blood pressure. I was feeling strong. He was still feeling strong. I feel like nothing is happening to him, no fever, no headache, but he say, 'How can a somebody like me be included in such a thing?' That he won't allow such a thing to happen. He said, 'The day the thing will occur on my body and people will just be watching me like this?'" She shook her head and looked away from me. "My husband, he stay just one year before he finally give up. Maybe he took something. I thought that he take something, because he was very healthy. He was very healthy. That's why I say he took something." She closed the album and replaced it beneath the table.

"So as I am now," she said after a long pause, "I'm not feeling any pains. The only thing that I do is to take my drugs. I started taking drugs two years ago. Two years ago, I force myself to take drugs. I just want it like that, because I feel that if I'm not taking the drugs, along the line I will break down or something like that. I take ARV. I'm living healthy. I watch the kind of food I eat. I place myself on vegetables, fruits, all these local-local foods—dry fish, crayfish. I just press myself on it. Then every month, I make sure I take malaria drugs. I deworm myself. If I stay something like three months, I will went to test and check my CD4 count. That's how I used to do."

She stretched and yawned, suddenly so casual, so ordinary.

Such is a reality of HIV/AIDS. It is an immensely transformative process that can dramatically change a life or lives—from prosperity to poverty, from popularity to a marginalized existence near the edge of a city. Yet the reality is that even with HIV, life can go on, and in the most boring of fashions. There may be a new normal to which one must adjust, but if that adjustment can be made, then chores must be completed, money must be earned, children must be cared for. There is nothing sexy or dramatic about a life lived normally. When considering HIV/AIDS, people want to see a dramatic change. They want to feel that they have rescued someone from the verge of death, but the reality of dealing with HIV/AIDS is as Rolake suggested, that effort should be put into making sure people maintain their level of existence. People from Nigeria and abroad don't want to hear that their donations and aid work are going to support another person's ability to do the things we all have to do, but this should be our goal in the struggle with HIV/AIDS: to mitigate its impact so that lives become livable again.

"The only thing I know is that as I am now, I'm not going to die because of this problem," Hope said to me shortly before we parted ways. "I know that this problem will not kill me. As of now," she said, "I find it like malaria. When malaria comes to you, you go to hospital and take drugs; it will stop. Instead of me to have cancer or diabetes, it is better I will be into this problem because it doesn't disturb me. Nothing. This is just like ordinary sickness."

STIGMA

B ut HIV/AIDS is not really an ordinary sickness. It is not a cold or the flu, which, though contagious, are rarely deadly. It is not cancer or diabetes or heart disease, which are long-term and debilitating, sometimes deadly but not contagious. This is not to downplay the significance of the epidemic but rather to suggest, as Philip Alcabes does in his essay "The Ordinariness of AIDS," that HIV/AIDS is extraordinary because it attracts so much attention from the global population, perhaps more than any other disease since the medieval plague. It causes intense fear, initially bordering on hysteria, which influences how we see both the disease and people who have it.

As long as there has been life, there have been viruses—or so I learned in medical school. Indeed, a virus might be a primitive form of existence. Viruses are inordinately simple creatures composed of genetic material, either DNA or RNA, surrounded by a protein shell. Their sole purpose is to replicate, to make more copies of themselves by inserting their genetic material into the genetic material of a host, such as a human cell, and making that cell generate more copies of the virus. We get sick because the virus often destroys our cells in the process of replicating itself.

In general, human immunodeficiency virus (HIV) behaves no differently from other viruses. It cannot survive on its own and must have a host organism to replicate itself and continue its life cycle. HIV is unique, however, because of the particular cell in the human body it chooses as its host. The virus's primary target is one of the most crucial cells for human survival, the helper T cell. These cells coordinate our immune system's response to most of the illnesses we might encounter during our lives. HIV makes millions of copies of itself inside the helper T cell and then destroys the cell to release all of its copies into the bloodstream. It is so devastating a pathogen because it attacks the body's ability to fight infection—including HIV itself.

AIDS (acquired immune deficiency syndrome) occurs when the HIV virus has destroyed so many helper T cells that our bodies can't begin to mount an immune response to even a simple illness. In other words, our bodies' immune system cells cannot talk to one another. They act in isolation, and we are left extremely vulnerable to infections our bodies wouldn't ordinarily sneeze at.

AIDS is not one illness but a constellation of sicknesses that can occur when our immune systems stop working. People with AIDS can get various forms of cancer, pneumonias, and fungal infections, along with bacterial and viral illnesses that our bodies might otherwise prevent. Because it takes a long time—on average about five years—for someone to lose enough helper T cells to progress to AIDS, a person with HIV may not look ill (in fact you can argue they are not ill) until the very last stages of HIV infection. It is just not possible to determine by looking who may or may not have HIV. This is perhaps one of the most important survival mechanisms for the virus. Because people who carry HIV do not necessarily appear sick, they are more likely to unknowingly pass the virus along to another person through the exchange of bodily fluids like blood, semen, or vaginal fluids. Thus, unlike other epidemics that announce themselves rather loudly, the HIV/AIDS epidemic is relatively silent.

HIV/AIDS is made all the more extraordinary because of the intersection of its biological and social effects. "In truth," Alcabes writes, "there is no clearly demarcated biological disease divorced from the social narrative of the epidemic. . . . No matter how sophisticated our molecular virology is (and it is, today) the virus is only part of the story of the epidemic." Dr. Chukwumuanya Igboekwu, known as Doc to his friends, would agree. His small organization, Physicians for Social Justice, operates in northern Nigeria to raise awareness about HIV/AIDS and provide services for people living with the disease. We first met in New York City on an unseasonably warm day for early March. I remember using my sweater sleeve to wipe away perspiration on my forehead after the brisk walk through a still barren Morningside Park and up the steps along its cliffs to Columbia University. Out of breath, I met Doc standing outside Nussbaum & Wu, a popular bagel shop and café, shivering in a large black winter down coat.

"I need to go home," he said. "Kai, this country is cold."

We laughed. His laugh was goofy for such a serious face, so much older than the twenty-seven years he had lived. He looks young, but his face appears thoroughly prepared for the most intense stress—a bus accident with forty casualties, a woman with a complicated pregnancy—and this gives him a sense of gravitas. After three years of friendship, I now understand. Since the age of twenty-five, Doc has been in a rural part of northern Nigeria, the lone doctor serving hundreds of thousands of people, whose language he does not speak and whose customs and religion he does not share. In his short career, he has seen nearly everything and learned to be prepared for anything.

According to Doc, the spread of a disease is not

just a biological event; it is also social. Our reactions to HIV/AIDS and our effectiveness at stopping its spread depend on preexisting social and political conditions that both inform and are informed by its presence in our societies.

"I remember the case of one police officer, a sergeant, my friend," Doc said above the buzz of conversation and spoons tinkling against coffee cups and pastry plates. "I didn't see him for some time, so I started asking, 'Where is this guy?' They said he was not feeling fine. I went to his house, and when I saw him, I was shocked. He has lost weight. He couldn't stand up again. I asked him, 'What is wrong with you?' The only thing he said is 'Doctor, they said it's AIDS.'" The policeman was in the end stages of AIDS, Doc told me. It didn't have to get this bad, but the community's ideas about AIDS had affected the progression of the police officer's disease.

Instead of seeking help, the sergeant had gone into seclusion because of his diagnosis, attempting to avoid contact with family, friends, and the community at large because of the negative opinions and community sanction that would result if people knew his diagnosis. Doc explained that he tried to mobilize for his friend, that he rushed to Minna, the capital of Niger State, about three hours south of where he lives and works, to get additional medicines like immune system boosters from the regional office of an international NGO, but it was too late. The sergeant's illness had progressed too far.

"By the time I came back, the guy had died. Just like that." He clasped his hands together on the table and let them rest around the cup of tea steaming in front of him. I sipped from my own.

"You know, I talked with his children." Doc's voice broke a little as he spoke. "Because later they came to collect his medical certificate. When I wrote the medical certificate for them, they didn't let me say it was HIV. I just told them he died of immunosuppressive disease. I didn't feel so bad because I was not lying outrightly. HIV is an immunosuppressive disease, but somebody that is not a medical guy wouldn't understand what that is. I do that a lot. There are some cases where they will not allow you to write HIV/AIDS. In fact, I don't think I've ever written HIV/AIDS. I never write HIV/AIDS. I always put immunosuppressive disease. You can write any other thing. You can write heart attack, hypertension, but they will not be happy if you write HIV as the cause of death, AIDS as the cause of death." The diagnosis of HIV/AIDS carries such weight that people are just as eager to avoid it in death as they are in life. No one wants to be a permanent outcast.

The sergeant's family left town soon after his

death. When Doc urged the man's wife to get tested for HIV, she refused.

"Why did she not want to get tested?" I asked, almost involuntarily.

The answer came later when I joined Doc in one of the rural northern Nigerian villages where he worked.

Sahon-Rami is a remote village in predominantly Muslim Niger State, five hours north of Nigeria's capital, Abuja—even at the speed Doc drives. He careened down the two-lane highways, passing large trucks when the road cleared, swerving to avoid potholes, and laughing as I gripped the passenger-door armrest in terror. He knows the roads well—where the police checkpoints usually pop up and when to hang his stethoscope from the rearview mirror so that the officers wouldn't stop us and ask for bribes. As we sped further north, the signs of human life grew more intermittent. Vast open fields of scraggly bush, occasionally broken by a large tree or accumulation of boulders, stretched from the road on either side. Sahon-Rami is a small community in the middle of one of these open expanses. With a spread-out group of other hamlets, it forms the Mashegu local government area, population two hundred thousand, most of whom are Doc's patients. Some of the areas are so remote that they are accessible only by motorbike. Even in Sahon-Rami, Doc joked, you need to climb a tree to get a signal on your mobile phone.

Once we got settled in his small house, down the road from the clinic where he worked, Doc took me to the village square, a small clearing to the side of Sahon-Rami's rough, red-earth main road. It was bordered on the other three sides by mud-brick houses capped with thatch or rusting corrugated tin roofing. A complement of tree stumps used as seats and smoothed by years of friction from the bottoms of villagers filled the otherwise open dusty space. Not far from us, little boys roughhoused in the meager shade of a bone-dry tree, climbing its branches in a diversion from the path between their lessons at school and their work in the fields. Little girls in various colors of headscarves walked one another home with much more order and purpose than their male counterparts. They stopped in groups before each low-standing mud-brick thatch-roofed house as their numbers slowly were whittled away. Here everyone knew everyone—indeed, many families were related by blood or marriage. Everybody also seemed to know everybody else's business—who did or didn't go to mosque, who did or didn't pitch in for the community grinding mill (which spewed thick black exhaust up and over a thatch fence), the births, the deaths, and all the usual stuff of rural community life.

It was here that I met Idris, a young self-proclaimed youth leader and community politician. Tall and lanky, he sported a red fez cap with a tassel he repeatedly waved away from his face. His long beige caftan had a ring of red dust around its lower hem. The same red dust covered his toes and leather sandals.

"Here? Now? If we are suspecting either man or woman, if you are suspecting that they have HIV, no one will come closer to you," he said when I asked him what people in the area thought about HIV/AIDS. "If you are a man, no woman will come closer to you. If you are a woman, no man will come closer to you. Everybody is afraid. You know community people now. Villagers—everybody does not want to lose his life."

I believed him. He seemed to know every inch of this community. Idris *had* to know this place. It was an election year, and he had spent countless hours on his motorbike or on foot traversing a vastness in which the politics, in addition to being about money, was about your family, your friends, and what they all thought of you. His community was small-village Nigeria, where the days roll over slowly and nothing seems to change.

"I remember some years ago," he told me. "One lady, they were suspecting her because she's very lean and she's always on bed—fever, all of this. We are suspecting maybe it's HIV. They banish her. They took her away. I don't know where they took her to. They only made sure she should leave the community."

He was evasive in answering my follow-up questions. What did she look like? Silence. Who pushed her out? "The youths."

Were you there? Silence—leaving me to imagine what a scene that might have been. What about her family, her protection? As I have been told, in some of these situations, the family is quick to abandon the ailing person. They give her a separate space in the compound, bring food and clear used dishes, but that is all. Conversation, a loving touch, reassurance— like health, these things all fade away in the face of HIV/AIDS. She would have been profoundly alone.

"Where did she go?" I asked him.

Idris was silent for a moment. He then said softly, "They made sure she should leave."

An older man overheard us speaking. He looked up from the prayer beads he was trying to string back together. He picked each one off the ground and threaded it down a long black piece of rope. Beads fell from the other end when he diverted his attention.

"Nobody can tell you that he has it," he chimed in. "If people knows that he has the disease, people will try to isolate themselves from him or her so that the disease will not be transmit."

This isolation that Doc, Idris, and the old man describe is the result of the unique stigma associated with HIV/AIDS. In his seminal work *Stigma*, the sociologist Erving Goffman defines stigma as a trait that can turn people away, an "undesired differentness from what we had anticipated." He argues that stigma comes in three distinct but related forms: abominations of the body, perceived blemishes of individual character, and the stigma of race, nation, or religion. Abominations of the body are physical deformities that set one apart. Blemishes of individual character are alleged moral, mental, or emotional flaws for which a person receives societal condemnation. Finally Goffman considers the stigma of race, nation, culture, or religion to be the result of inheritable traits that can be passed along and shared as a result of affiliation.

Stigma has enjoyed a lasting relationship with disease. In general, disease usually associates the carrier with one or perhaps two of Goffman's three manifestations of stigma. For example, the lepers of biblical and medieval times were cast aside because of their unsightly bacteria-eaten flesh. In the present day, heart disease can sometimes be a stigmatizing illness because it is associated with gluttony and sloth. The stigma of HIV/AIDS, however, is more profound and complicated because it combines all three categories of stigma and so brands the victim and associated community not once but three times over.

If abominations of the body are a form of stigma, then HIV/AIDS in its end stages causes plenty. Most of my exposure to the stigmata of HIV/AIDS

occurred while I was on the AIDS care team at Columbia University during my third and fourth years
of medical school, and I would often find it hard to
observe the physical deterioration of some of the patients we cared for. I remember one woman who
suffered from persistent and painful *Candida* fungal
infections of her mouth and throat. Each morning,
despite treatment with antifungal mouthwashes and
scrubbing with a toothbrush, she would have a thick
white film at the back of her throat, on her tongue,
cheeks, and lips. Another patient I helped to care for
came to the hospital with the multiple itching, ooz-
ing sores of *prurigo nodularis,* which can sometimes
occur in patients with HIV. These lesions made it
impossible for him to lie comfortably in bed, so he
squirmed and scratched constantly, picking at old
scabs and opening new weeping wounds that glis-
tened in the harsh overhead light. Other patients I
saw suffered from persistent diarrhea or the AIDS-
related cancer Kaposi's sarcoma, which can cause dis-
figuring red tumors to form on a patient's skin. They
were clearly marked by their illnesses in ways that
were hard to ignore.

I found it difficult not to be overwhelmed by the
physical presentation of some of our patients. The
desire to recoil and protect oneself is not admirable,
but it can be so strong that at first it can be hard to

see beyond the manifestations of a disease, to see that before you lies a person with a disease—not a disease with a person. I would often marvel to myself while I stood outside a patient's bedroom as I put on gloves and a protective gown, and after as I lathered my hands with sanitizer—standard hospital procedure to protect both patients and care providers—how thin this line is between professional responsibility and fear. If I and others with a background in health and knowledge of how HIV/AIDS works and is transmitted can be shocked by its physical signs, what to do then if you are a villager in a rural area without much information beyond the idea that HIV/AIDS is bad? What do you do if you witness a friend, as one man recalled to me, with "her whole body fill up with sores. Her skin color just change from yellow to black like that."

What makes HIV/AIDS even more disconcerting is the fact that a diagnosis is still often considered a death sentence. Idris explained to me that in Hausa-speaking northern Nigeria, the word for HIV/AIDS is *kanjamau*. This translates roughly as "skeleton." In addition to suggesting the emaciated physical appearance of a person with HIV/AIDS, it also brings to mind the ultimate abomination of the human physical form, the stuff of horror films and nightmares, the living dead. If being negative is ordinary, then this HIV-positive person languishing in this liminal state, not quite alive, not yet dead, is clearly abnormal and as such suffers from discrimination that can lead to isolation and neglect.

However, the nature of this disease is that it often does not show for years. This complicates its associated stigma. "You can't see it because it doesn't written for anybody's face," the old man in Idris's village square said. He was expressing a common sentiment: you can't see it, so be afraid. In other words, now more than ever we must use vigilance and segregate ourselves from these dangerous HIV-infected Others, even if, paradoxically, we cannot immediately recognize their difference.

The disease is also seen as a commentary on a person's moral standing. As one doctor I spoke with briefly about HIV put it, "Whenever people see you, they say, 'Oh! Here is a sinner—somebody must have gone and done something really bad.' People don't want to be associated with that." Thus HIV causes a remarkable metamorphosis, making the extrinsic and physical an intrinsic property of character. An HIV-positive person becomes at best a person with flawed judgment and at worst someone evil.

"Dearly beloved, it has pleased God to afflict you

with this disease, and the Lord is gracious for bringing punishment upon you for the evil that you have done in this world"—Michel Foucault quotes from a French ritual when discussing the treatment of lepers in medieval times. He might as well have described the present attitude toward those with HIV/AIDS, in Nigeria and perhaps elsewhere in the world. Despite the increasing availability of scientific information about the nature of HIV transmission, there are still many Nigerians who believe the disease is punishment for individual sins and aggregate societal ills. The anthropologist Daniel Jordan Smith has studied Nigerian attitudes toward HIV/AIDS and found that "the dominant religious discourse about AIDS is that it is a scourge visited by God on a society that has turned its back on religion and morality." He recalls conversations with HIV-positive Nigerians who attributed their disease to the "sinful immoral lives they had led."

The impact of such thinking can be devastating. An HIV-positive woman I met briefly on a trip to Lagos explained to me the personal impact of this kind of moralizing on HIV infection.

"Even in church, *my church*, then, they saw it as a big taboo," she said. "The way the man would be preaching and be saying things: 'We're telling people don't be a prostitute when you're young. You should behave well. You should have good upbringing.' I felt he was passing the wrong information because I, as far as I am concerned, I had a good upbringing. I wouldn't justify that I was a saint, but I know that to a great extent I had a very good upbringing. I felt that man was passing the wrong information. That information was scary. He was putting the immediate society in a tight corner because among the people there, you wouldn't tell me that I was the only one who was positive in that church. You can imagine the wrong information that he might be sending to that man or that woman who is HIV positive— that you are a prostitute! You are a bad person! He was being too judgmental, so you go home judging yourself to death: 'Oh! I'm a bad person. I don't even deserve to live in this world anymore. Oh! Nothing good can come out of me.' Those were the messages that were always surrounding the pastor's message, the message of death, judgment, guilt, failure." She stressed the word *prostitute* each time, almost spat it out at me with vehemence as if trying to clear her mouth of something bad-tasting.

The relationship between HIV and sexuality is complex and deserves special consideration. A major aspect of the moral component of HIV-related stigma derives from our anxieties about sex. Again, the work of Daniel Jordan Smith is instructive. His interviews with young Nigerians on the subject of sexual morality and HIV/AIDS yielded comments like "AIDS is God's way of checking the immoral sexual behavior that is rampant in Nigeria now." The intense focus on sexual impropriety as a cause for both the existence and the spread of HIV/AIDS leads to the conclusion that the moral failings of an individual can endanger society as a whole, making it all the more important to brand and exclude fallen individuals—to prevent additional lapses and mitigate the impact of those that have already occurred. Unfortunately, this practice can backfire, because it drives frank discussion about the nature of HIV to the margins and discourages honesty about diagnoses for fear of judgment and stigmatization. It creates a silence that facilitates the spread of the disease.

Finally and perhaps most dramatically, the physical and moral forms of stigma associated with HIV/ AIDS attach not only to individuals but also to racial groups, countries, in fact a whole continent—Africa. The locus of the worst manifestations of the HIV/ AIDS epidemic in sub-Saharan Africa reinforces preexisting stigmatizing notions of Africans as inferior and Africa as a backward place. Ideas about Africans and Africa as unacceptably different are long-standing and complicated, and they have already been explored by many writers and thinkers. Africans have traditionally been considered emotionally and intellectually inferior, our savage bodies finding purpose only when subordinated to the white man's will. During the colonial period, myths of savagery, ungodly ritual, human sacrifice, and profligate sexuality became more common as an increasingly violent subjugation of the colonized necessitated ever more imaginative justifications. Some have argued that the branding of Africans as inferior emerged as exploitation of Africa's natural resources, including African bodies as cheap labor, increased. In other words, in order to legitimize the abuse of another human, colonial masters had to diminish the humanity of their subjects and emphasize the otherness of the place from which they came.

Anthropological and scientific writings of the colonial period are shot through with these sentiments. Among the more precise—and prescient—is Joseph Conrad's fictional work about the Congo, *Heart of Darkness*. Conrad connected African inferiority and disease in a way that anticipated present-day racial and cultural stigmatization of those with HIV/AIDS in Africa:

> Black shapes crouched, lay, sat between the trees leaning against the trunks, clinging to the earth, half coming out, half effaced with the dim light, in all the attitudes of pain, abandonment and despair . . . they were

nothing earthly now—nothing but black
shadows of disease and starvation, lying con-
fusedly in the greenish gloom.

Conrad's Africans begin as feeble creatures too
weak to hold themselves up, too racked by the mis-
fortunes that their blackness has bestowed upon them
to stand tall and act with agency. They end as quasi-
humans, of another world, their forms merged fully
with disease and despair generated in the bowels
of a continent composed of primeval otherworldli-
ness. It is a testament to Conrad's descriptive genius
and literary influence, and unfortunately also to the
strength of the associations he so vividly captures,
that present descriptions of HIV/AIDS in Africa stray
very little from this script.

"Soon Africa will be a continent of AIDS orphans," begins CNN's former chief international
correspondent Christiane Amanpour in that television network's 2006 documentary *Where Have All the
Parents Gone?* A musical score of mournful reed flutes
plays as a map of Africa appears on screen, emphasizing the exotic otherness of the continent. There follows an image of young "African" (in reality, Kenyan)
children lolling in the dust as a baby cries and heavy
breathing interspersed with despondent moaning is
amplified over Amanpour's voice.

Next we are introduced to Mukhtar, who we are informed is "another African boy who wonders whether he too will become one of the million AIDS orphans in Kenya." The camera zooms in on his face while he watches his cachectic HIV-positive father breathing laboriously in bed. As Amanpour narrates Africa's struggle with AIDS, the screen fills with images of shabbily dressed people in shantytowns shrouded by red dust. Later we learn that Mukhtar's father, who was rejected by his family once they discovered his HIV-positive status, had considered killing himself, his wife, and his son with rat poison because they are "a burden" and he does not "want them to suffer." This snippet of a modern HIV/AIDS film echoes Conrad at his best, playing up that which sets Africa and Africans apart. Never mind that there is no monolithic African identity; Kenyans stand for all Africans. They live in otherworldly dwellings surrounded by filth. They even have a different, warped sense of morality. We are left wondering what kind of creature would consider killing not only himself but also his young wife and only son—of course, a person "infected with HIV." This is all before anyone questions whether it is ethical to display a young Kenyan boy with HIV-positive parents for millions of people to see. One wonders whether a white European or American child would have received the same treatment.

If this was but one representation, it might be ex-cusable, but it falls into a panoply of images of HIV/ AIDS in Africa that play up stigmatizing identifiers. As recently as 2006, the *New York Times* displayed headlines screaming "Traditional Ways Spread AIDS in Africa, Experts Say," deliberately evoking thoughts of strange ritual and exotic practices. We later find that one of these "traditional" ways is the universal practice of breastfeeding. Associations like this re-mind me of the poster I own from the AIDS charity Keep a Child Alive. Their public relations campaign unwittingly plays to ideas of African otherness while cementing the link between African-ness and HIV/ AIDS. In this image, the two are inextricably linked. Disease is African-ness and African-ness is a disease. So powerful is this association that a condition at-tributable to approximately 4 percent of the African continent's population becomes the narrative for the other 96 percent. It results in the following conclu-sions relayed to me by a young Canadian woman working in Lagos, who described the reactions of her family members to her decision to move to Nigeria for a year: "My dad's mom, when she found out I was going, she said, 'You're going to catch AIDS.' I had an aunt who told me that I should bring a bag of my own blood with me . . . if I needed a blood transfusion."

A *New Yorker* article about the possible origins of a theoretical next big epidemic consolidates the associations of African-ness with strange or backward culture and disease. It follows a Stanford University virologist who is desperately trying to educate local villagers about the perils of consuming monkeys because they are receptacles for disease. "When I see a monkey like that, dragged through the street, bloody, on the way to market, it's like looking at a loaded weapon," he says after seeing a woman carrying a monkey on the back of a motorcycle. The piece features Cameroonians covered in buckets of monkey blood and stresses that in the present day, with easy travel linkages between Cameroon and California, it's not hard for a virus to move between populations. This article is a striking example of what the medical anthropologist and AIDS activist Dr. Paul Farmer calls a "symbolic network that stresses exoticism and the endemicity of disease." In other words, diseases like HIV/AIDS come from people with "weird" or "backward" cultural practices—Africans who eat monkeys.

HIV/AIDS was not always associated primarily with Africa. Thirty years ago, the initial concerns about the virus were decidedly localized to the Western world. Homosexual men were initially vilified as the prime culprits for the propagation of the epidemic. At some point during the mid-1990s, when it became clear that there was an epidemic in Africa primarily spread by heterosexual sex, and when it became clear that public health programs along with readily available treatment in the West had led to a stabilization and decline in the number of new cases there, AIDS became African. That Africans in countries like Nigeria have not managed to control the spread of HIV/AIDS, as has been achieved in developed nations, supposedly reflects a host of vices for which Africans are constantly berated. We are disorganized and inefficient, so the virus spreads. We lack the intellectual capacity to create our own drugs and treatment protocols, so the virus spreads. We are untrustworthy and misappropriate funds for treatment programs, so the virus spreads. We lack compassion for the afflicted, so people die. In what might be the most unfortunate of ironies, we are stigmatized for stigmatizing: that is, according to the narrative, in developed nations people are cared for; they are not ostracized; they receive services and treatment. In Africa the infected, like Mukhtar's father, are savagely expelled—as if fear of contagion is a uniquely African sentiment—cast out into the vast darkness of a physically and morally undeveloped continent. This is not to say fear and stigma do not exist, but they are not uniquely African phenomena.

HIV/AIDS is an extraordinary illness, especially because it creates a social dynamic that in some ways mimics the biological process by which the HIV virus damages the human body. In the same way that the HIV virus causes a breakdown in communication among elements of our immune systems, leading to an inability to neutralize it and other diseases, so too does its associated stigma break down relationships among people, preventing many of those who have it from communicating their need for assistance and treatment. Indeed, a former senior World Health Organization (WHO) AIDS program official described stigma as a stage of the HIV/AIDS epidemic, "the stage of social impact . . . marked by stigma, grinding down its victims with shame and isolation, creating an environment of secrecy and denial which are both catalysts for HIV transmission." If to be open about one's status is to don a set of scarlet letters that says "not one of us," not human, then it is understandable why so many would remain silent about or ignorant of their status. The more the virus spreads, the more people die, and the stronger the stigma grows.

For me the impact of this stigma didn't really hit home until after a discussion I had with a young woman I met at a bar on a military base about an hour away from the village where Doc worked and lived. We decided to make a trip to the Nigerian Army cantonment one afternoon for a drink. Because the area is predominantly Muslim and governed in part by Sharia law, the military barracks, with its multicultural, multireligious makeup of soldiers from all over the country, was the only place to get a drink, a cold beer, maybe even a rudimentary cocktail. The environment was perfect for the large army base, which was home to an infantry and artillery unit. There were acres of open field for firing ranges and target practice. A sleepy barracks with one- and two-story living quarters in strict rows occupied one corner of the base. The officers' quarters were in another section nearby. Between them was an open-air space with multiple bars where young women served drinks and heaping plates of food to soldiers in fatigues. That's where I met Elizabeth. She was a server at one of the bars.

I can't remember exactly how our conversation started, but it turned quickly—as many of my conversations then did—to the subject of HIV/AIDS. Elizabeth was eager to talk. We agreed to meet later at a hotel where I was to stay the night so that we could talk with greater privacy.

Later that night, Elizabeth said, "I've gotten a sister," meaning a close friend. "She stopped the drugs

and she died. I never knew that she has been hiding."
We sat on the concrete veranda outside my guest
chalet just before dusk. The hotel compound was full
of similar chalets, simple concrete boxes surrounded
by small grassy gardens fenced by small shrubs. A few
stray chickens pecked at the gravel path for insects
hiding between the pebbles. There were two WHO
trucks parked beneath a red-blossomed flamboyant
tree. I would find out the next morning that they
belonged to two older British men managing a polio
eradication campaign.

The receding sunlight lingered on Elizabeth's
face. Her full cheeks had followed her from child-
hood into her twenties, and a rather delicate and un-
imposing nose appeared almost as an afterthought
between them. She wore dark eye shadow. Earlier,
at the bar, I had watched her move gracefully from
table to table serving drinks, seemingly flowing despite the long, tight purple skirt that forced her to
take small steps.

Her friend, Elizabeth told me, had been an excel-
lent tailor. For that reason, Elizabeth had encouraged
her to come up north to this town near the military
barracks, where there was more work. Arrangements
were made, and her friend soon journeyed from Cross
River to Niger State to set up shop, start sewing, and
hopefully earn some money. Her friend wasn't to stay

for very long. "Her mom died and she travel home," Elizabeth said. "Later, I went home because I lost a cousin's sister. When I saw my friend, she was down. I sympathized for her sickness and everything. Something swell her under the chest there," Elizabeth said. She placed her palm flat against the right side of her stomach.

"I don't know the problem. I was always asking her, and she said she don't know. She don't know. When she came back to us," up north, "I took her to so many labs. They said she has a liver problem, that her liver has been affected like that. So I now send her with my other sister to my pastor that they should go for prayers. I call on the pastor. I said, 'Please, my sister is coming for prayers. She's not well. If she come, please interview her and ask her if she's gone for tests. It's not as if you're suspecting her, but tell her: go test for this HIV thing, that you may be sick.'

"The man of God now ask her those questions. The man of God even assisted, gave her a thousand naira, and we went to the lab and did the test. That day they did her the HIV test, she was afraid when she came out. She didn't want us to know. The lab man said there are signs of HIV, that we will come back and do the test maybe in a month or three months later, but that she should first go and treat that liver problem.

"I was afraid. I now had to call and tell this girl's father that she is sick and I wouldn't want any bad thing to happen and have them say I kept her here. But the first question the father asked me is 'Has she dropped her drugs?'

"I said, 'Which drugs, Papa?'

"'She didn't tell you she has a problem?' he asked.

"The man now explained everything to me, that she has been on AIDS drug, that maybe she drops the drugs and that's why she has been sick. He said I should send her home."

The darkness had stolen over us slowly as we sat chatting. It was night now and there was no electricity. I could see glowing orange hurricane lanterns floating through the night as the hotel staff crunched across the gravel while winding up the evening cleaning. Quicker steps could be heard across the path in front of us to a hulking building that housed the hotel's diesel generator. There was a click followed by a sputtering low rumble, then light.

"I never knew that she has been hiding, pretending that she was afraid of the result. So I question her that morning: 'How long did you stop taking HIV drugs? When did you last collect them?' She said she collected lastly three months ago. Then for two months she has not taken the drugs. That is why she is down. So they took her back home. I was told that they went and did her CD4 count test and other test. But later we still lost her. That is how HIV kill."

Elizabeth's face was heavy with pain. Her mind seemed tortured by the same questions that left me unsettled. Why had her friend kept up this ruse, gone for multiple tests, and feigned nervousness in anticipation of a result she already knew? Could she have been hoping for some miraculous change that would render her normal again, that would remove the disease that had her living undercover? Why such elaborate deception? Elizabeth will never know, but the likelihood is that the stigma associated with HIV/AIDS forced her friend to hide her illness and possibly to discontinue the care that would have kept her alive.

"It's not everyone that will see you having that problem that will be embracing you," Elizabeth said after some time. "It's not everybody that will embrace you back—even your sisters in the house. You understand? Even in the village of my sister that died, many people were saying it: 'Sure say no be AIDS?' Even the old ones were saying, 'Abeg oh! We hear say nah [it is] AIDS. If nah AIDS, make she die. Make she no come distribute.' Old women! They were saying it."

She spat with disgust.

"I have a little sister, a friend, that was staying

with us. She wasn't drinking in the same cup that my sister who died was drinking. If we put soup together, she will not eat. She was always selecting the spoons so as not to share spoon that my sister was using. Even when she never heard of it being HIV, she suspected that it should be that. Two of them were best friends, but see, when one was sick, the other could not show that love. She was keeping her far from herself." Elizabeth shook her head and raised her fingers to massage her cheeks. "So HIV prevent love. It cut relationship of love."

HIV/AIDS-related stigma severs the connection that one person forms with another. It is so strong that it can even make speaking out about the disease problematic.

"You are the first person I am telling that my sister died on that," Elizabeth mumbled to me. Her chin dropped to her chest. "But if I use her own example to help somebody, that is, by telling the person that, 'See, my sister have died on this thing. Please!' I don't think that God will punish me for that. I know that God will have mercy on me that I am not abusing my sister.

"I want to talk to people concerning this thing. Me, I wanted even to stand in my village and at least arrange the women, the men, or the youth—all of them—and discuss it with them: 'See this thing that you people are saying about this girl. Many of you, you have not been tested. Many of you have it. It may be killing some women, married women, they will not know! One two, one two they die. You won't know if it is HIV.' That is what I wanted to do. That is what I have determined in my mind because I feel that people are dying in that village and they don't know what is killing them. Maybe it might be AIDS that is killing them and there are drugs to prevent the thing. Another of my sister said, 'No! Before you will start saying those things, they will say we done carry am.'" Elizabeth sighed and crossed her arms. "I just left. They buried her, and I just left. I left."

Elizabeth's friend need not have died. But HIV/ AIDS has such power that it can cut people off from one another, leaving those who most need support isolated and vulnerable. Its stigma and the result- ing fear of abandonment and discrimination make extremely difficult a greater openness that can help treat its symptoms and prevent its spread. An ordi- nary sickness does not cause so fraught and convo- luted a reaction.

Elizabeth stopped speaking. We sat together on the warm concrete, our bodies separated by two bottles of Coke I had retrieved from the fridge in my room. Insects buzzed about the fluorescent light above us, their shadows floating across our bodies.

Somewhere beyond the hotel compound, the highway pulsed with the horns of tractor-trailers warning cars, motorcycles, and pedestrians as they sped down an unlit road.

"When I think about my sister, I feel it very well," she said after some time. "There is no day I don't think about her since I lost her. There is a place we worshiped together where there's a particular lady that sings 'Everything You Find Is in Jesus.' If you find money, that it's in Jesus; if you find health, it's in Jesus; if you find life, it's in Jesus. If they pray such prayers or sing such chorus now, I really feel. I will be in the church crying. I cry for her own. I do feel her. I've not forgotten about her. I feel her very well.

"I shed tear for my sister each time when I see people surviving with this thing. In fact, when I was sick with ulcer, I went to Nnamdi Azikiwe Teaching Hospital, and if you see the lineup of people with HIV to collect drugs, that's why I say, 'How can you just lost your life like that?' You understand? Because people go there and take drugs free! Then how will you just stay and lost your life like that? I don't think God has designed that she has to die. She doesn't have to died."

SEX

I'm actually going to a brothel, I remember thinking as my friend Doc and I drove to a truck stop about an hour west of his village clinic. He had set up services there for a number of sex workers patronized by the intercity truck drivers who stopped for a few hours' rest. At the truck stop, fields of tall brown grass and low shrubs stretched outward from the junction and its impromptu settlement of zinc-roofed, mud-brick buildings. Around us large trucks rested as their engines clicked while cooling and their drivers propped themselves against their large tires or in the shade beneath their chassis. The men were almost catatonic from a full day's work of driving. Their only motions were to raise plastic cups of water to their lips. Not too far away, a line of women sat silently against a low cement wall, some of them eating roasted corn, others fanning themselves against the heat.

"Those women are sex workers," Doc said, thrusting his chin in their general direction.

The year before, during the Nigerian gubernatorial elections, I had interviewed a local Lagos politician about Nigeria's HIV/AIDS epidemic. During our meeting in his dimly lit office, he had suggested that the disease was a problem of interstate truck drivers and female sex workers.

"For instance," he had said, "a tanker driver is supposed to leave from Lagos all the way to Kano to deliver fuel. Because of the kind of person he is—he's very promiscuous—he stops at Ore. He has a 'friend' in Ore, and let's say he picks the HIV virus up in Ore along the way. He's infected. From Ore, he now gets to Lokoja, where he's also promiscuous. There he has unprotected sex with somebody, casual sex. He leaves. He has infected a community there. He gets all the way to Kano, where he has another show and a shot of it, casual sex again. He has infected someone in Kano. Then from Kano he heads back again to Lokoja and Abuja, and the person he had sex with is not available at that point in time, so he has sex with another person. A single carrier can do such damage. Along the routes of transportation, different cells and communities of infected people begin to spread."

I found his words interesting because they seemed to externalize both the epidemic and its primary means of transmission—sex. By focusing on these groups of people that Nigerians traditionally consider promiscuous or of lax morality, he seemed to suggest that normal people with normal monogamous sexual relationships exist outside the reach of the virus. Or as one woman I interviewed, who had recently graduated from college, put it: "Everybody wants to believe that they're very good and they're too clean for all of that; that people that die of AIDS or have HIV are dirty people, people that sleep around or do rubbish and stuff, not our kind of people."

"Some of them are positive," Doc said about the sex workers. He had just started offering testing and counseling services to the women along with education on safe sex practices and free condoms. The previous week, he said, some of the women had tested positive.

As we stood watching, every so often a man would walk toward the women and the pair would disappear through a nondescript door in the side of a low cement wall. It was almost too perfect. It seemed that right before my eyes, this politician's theory was being borne out.

I followed Doc across the street to that same narrow door in the side of the wall. He opened it and we stepped inside. Behind the door was a labyrinth of corridors open to the sky with smooth concrete walls broken at regular intervals by metal doors, some shut tight, others covered by limp and grungy curtains. At the end of one corridor, a youngish woman swept rhythmically, stopping every so often to slam the head of her broom against the ground and even out its bristles of stiff, dried grass before starting her motion again. Otherwise it was silent. I'm not sure what noises I expected, maybe even wished to hear in some realm of my imagination—heavy breathing, moaning, the universal indicators of illicit activity. But there was nothing. There was no intrigue here, no color, no vibrancy—just a bunch of dark rooms, each with a mattress and neatly arranged personal effects at its base.

At the end of one corridor, Doc introduced me to two women he had come to know very well through his advocacy work. His words were quick and almost apologetic: "This is my friend. He has come to do research on HIV. Can he ask you some questions?" Then he disappeared into the maze of corridors.

My new companions sat down on low stools in the corridor, their backs supported by the cement wall. I took a stool facing them and stretched out my legs as they had.

One of the women puffed her cheeks wide before smiling at me. She was naturally radiant, the woman at the party who makes everyone feel comfortable and looked after. She wore a red and orange rappa (a sari-like garment) wound around her legs and torso. The knot holding up the fabric sat in the dead center of a bright red T-shirt stretched tightly over her chest. A black scarf covered her hair. Her companion was a darker-complexioned woman with wrinkled skin on her fingers, her exposed arms, and in the corners of her lips and eyes that made her look like the peel of a desiccated yam. She didn't say much except to chime in for emphasis.

Our conversation began rather benignly with the usual pleasantries, after which the women shared with me their comprehensive knowledge of HIV/AIDS.

"We were taught," the first woman said at one point. "We went to lectures with the doctors, and they told us there is a tablet for it, but it cannot cure. This tablet can only subdue the various diseases. This is the worst disease we have in Nigeria. If you pregnant, then it will affect the baby."

"The worst!" her companion agreed.

But things changed dramatically when, in an attempt to shift the conversation, I asked softly, "How many men do you see in a day?"

Immediately the woman wearing the red shirt changed. Her natural ruddiness paled. Her smile became synthetic. The second woman sucked in her teeth with disapproval. "That question has no answer," she responded. "This is a road. Million of men can pass here in a day."

"Why do you ask?" the first lady said. "There is no need of that."

Why did I ask? It almost certainly doesn't matter what the numbers are, except for what asking about them suggests. It has taken me some reflection to truly understand the significance of my question—indeed, my whole interaction with these two women—especially within the larger context of the HIV/AIDS epidemic and its relation to sex. The primary issue that has concerned me for some time is why I felt the need to start my exploration of the relationship between HIV/AIDS and sex with sex workers. With 35.6 percent of sex workers in Nigeria testing positive for HIV, there is surely some epidemiological justification for doing so, but if I am honest, there is something else at play, subtly expressed in my supposedly innocent question about how many men each woman was to see that day. It is the same sentiment that caused the politician to associate the HIV/AIDS epidemic solely with the sexual practices of prostitutes and truck drivers. It is the same sentiment that initially led some to look at the scope of the HIV/AIDS epidemic in Africa and suggest that if, as Susan Sontag has put it, "AIDS is understood as a disease not only of sexual excess but of perversity," then Africans must be more promiscuous and perverse than the general population. This desire to define a type of sex or sexuality that is more closely associated with HIV/AIDS, followed by an overt or implied judgment about the newly defined group, probably speaks more to society's general anxiety about sex and sexual morality than it does to the practices of the group in question. This anxiety about sex has affected how we consider sexual relationships during the HIV/AIDS epidemic.

From the time of its appearance, HIV/AIDS has been linked with the idea of an unnatural or morally transgressive sexuality. It divided the public into those who have HIV or are at higher risk of contracting the virus and what Sontag called "*this* disease's version of 'the general population': white heterosexuals who do not inject themselves with drugs or have sexual relations with those who do." The appearance of HIV helped to enforce the idea of a normative sexuality exemplified and practiced by white men and women, all sex outside of this realm receiving the label *abnormal* or, still worse, *dangerous*.

When HIV first appeared in homosexual populations in the United States in the early 1980s, it was thought that something intrinsic to gay sex was the cause of both the virus and its spread. The medical literature contained references to GRID (gay-related immune deficiency), which then morphed into the popularly used "gay plague." In the late 1980s, massive efforts to educate the public about HIV/AIDS and strong campaigns by gay-rights advocates drastically reduced the presence of such dehumanizing rhetoric in the West. But rather than disappearing, the connection between HIV/AIDS and "weird" sex simply changed geographical locus as the extent of the sub-Saharan epidemic revealed itself.

The idea of African sexuality as Other in international dialogue begins first with accounts of Arab and Portuguese explorers in precolonial times. Themes of sexual aggressiveness, promiscuity, and strange sexual rituals addressed first in these early accounts have attached themselves to the sexualities of African and black peoples, coloring commentary on the subject for the greater part of the past millennium. Some have suggested that such accounts reflect the projections of European men from societies where the sexual experience was considered to be more strictly governed by explicitly understood social or religious convention, that the fascination and disgust with a perceived limitless African sexuality encountered on the frontier was the result of frustrated sexual expression at home.

More recently such themes have surfaced in the context of the African HIV/AIDS epidemic. For some both on and off the continent, the widespread presence of HIV/AIDS in Africa confirms that there is indeed something untoward about the way Africans approach sex. I am reminded of an encounter I had a few years ago while passing through London on my way back to Abuja when I decided to delay my onward journey by a couple of days to catch up with an old college friend. On a warmish spring evening, after dinner, we found ourselves in front of a nightclub discussing the only thing I seemed able to talk about—HIV. I was just explaining to my friend how prevalence rates in Nigeria—indeed, throughout much of Africa—had recently been downwardly revised, when the attractive young woman in a black blazer, skinny jeans, and heels standing in front of us turned around, a tad tipsy, and asked, "Isn't HIV the disease that started because someone in Africa had sex with a monkey?" While that statement can initially be dismissed as the silly musing of an ignorant drunk woman, it does reflect a line of thinking that was found in scholarly literature about HIV/AIDS in Africa. Consider this observation by the medical anthropologist Daniel Hrdy—which might be considered one of the more benign explanations for the origin and spread of HIV/AIDS in Africa:

> Although generalizations are difficult, most traditional African societies are promiscuous by Western standards. . . .
> There is a striking analogy between promiscuity as a risk factor in humans and the

"promiscuous" behavior of vervets. Typi-
cally, female vervets, unlike baboons, are
sexually receptive for long periods . . . and
during that time mate with multiple male
partners, sometimes engaging in dozens of
copulations on a single day. . . .

We are left to conclude that even if HIV/AIDS
isn't the result of some African having sex *with* a
monkey, it has certainly spread because Africans
were having sex *like* monkeys.

This initial argument that the HIV/AIDS epidemic was the result of a base African sexuality was
rounded off in papers like "The Social Context of
AIDS in Sub-Saharan Africa," published by the anthropologists John and Pat Caldwell, which suggested
the spread of HIV/AIDS was linked to societies
where "virtue is related more to success in reproduction than to limiting profligacy," and the fact that
"polygyny exists on a scale not found in the Eurasian
system." It is useful to start with polygamy when discussing the HIV/AIDS epidemic because the reactions to this cultural practice and its implication in
the spread of the epidemic provide a starting point
for exploring understandings of the relationship between sex and HIV/AIDS in Nigeria.

Polygamy has long been a point of concern when

the world considers African sexuality—if indeed such a thing even exists. During the height of the British colonial project, it was thought that the "greatest struggle is not so much with heathenism and fetishness as with worldliness, unchristian marriages and polygamy." The assumption made in anthropological assessments such as the Caldwells' of the relationship of an aberrant African sexuality to HIV/AIDS is that polygamy institutionalizes an innate promiscuity that is central to the spread of disease. It is not difficult to see why earlier researchers came to this conclusion—especially considering the historical and anthropological bias favoring the idea of the promiscuous African. It also reveals why many Africans initially pushed so hard against the idea that HIV was actually a problem. No one wanted to really answer the question: what does it mean if these historians and anthropologists are right? Unfortunately, both the unfounded assumptions about African sexuality and the pushback against these assumptions colored the debate and perhaps delayed the formation of an effective strategy to deal with HIV/AIDS.

I didn't originally intend to explore the role of polygamy in the spread of the epidemic, but it came up in a conversation I had with the prominent activist Samaila Garba, who runs Amana, an association of people living with HIV/AIDS in the northern Nigerian town of Kontangora.

I first met Samaila when Doc and I passed through Kontangora on our way to the village where Doc had his clinic. Samaila lived on a busy street near the center of town, just behind the emir's sprawling palace compound, where kids kicking a soccer ball scurried to the roadside every time a car or motorcycle buzzed by and people made slow progress in their amblings, stopping every five minutes to greet another person they knew. Residences were indistinguishable from storefronts—goods for sale hung from or sat on almost every available hook and flat surface. People blinked repeatedly when stepping from the shade of their dwellings into the harsh, hot sun. Samaila emerged from his low doorway slightly stooped, but soon unfolded himself to his true height. He towered over most people, and with his bald head, dark skin, and chiseled facial features, he appeared the emblem of seriousness, a distinguished look that vanished as soon as his face exploded into an enthusiastic, toothy smile.

He was an unlikely activist. The son of a poor farmer, he had grown up in northern Nigeria with dreams of attending college and becoming, as he called it, a "big man." But due to the relative poverty of his family, he was not able to continue his education beyond secondary school. Instead he became a schoolteacher and later, after some persuasion by close friends, a police officer. He worked instructing new recruits on the intricacies of the law, and sometimes went undercover to break syndicates of livestock thieves operating in the vast farm and grazing lands of the north. He certainly fit the part of a police officer—his imposing presence and assured movements, his gestures controlled and authoritative, his voice at once calm and commanding. And though police officers in Nigeria are much maligned for petty corruption, he was unapologetic in his love for his former profession. "Whatever they say about policemen," he had told me when we first met, "I know it built my character. It made me strong. It taught me courage, and I believe that courage is what I brought along into this HIV/AIDS work that I am doing."

When next we met, it was at the Kontangora General Hospital, where the Amana Association had its headquarters. We met in a stuffy office that was filled with files detailing potential grants, stacked piles of community activism training manuals, and peer-counseling and testing brochures. Dust collected on an old, clearly unused computer beside which rested a picture of Samaila meeting the Queen of England. We took two plastic chairs outside to the shade of a large mango tree abutting the building, where a group of women, members of the association, sat across from us against the wall of the hospital ward, their legs stretched out on the dusty concrete before them, laughing and chatting as little gusts of wind made their headscarves ripple. Every so often, they glanced toward us and whispered.

"In 2001 I did accept that I was HIV positive. I made statements as such in the public," Samaila said, once we were seated. "It was quite a revolutionary thing to do in the north because nobody had done that before. It was very tough for myself and for the remaining members of my family. It affected my children. They became very despondent, first of all because their mother was lost. Then they were not happy at school—people were giving them a lot of headache. Their peers were giving them a lot of headache. They would tell them, 'Your father is Mr. AIDS! Your father is Mr. AIDS!' And my kids would cry their way back home. I found a lot of rejection from my immediate community. When I went for prayer in the mosques—even to pray in the mosques—people didn't want to stand by me," he said, still wounded.

"But I also knew and I saw that people were misinterpreting the issue of HIV/AIDS. And I realized that the onus of removing the stigma lies on me and me only. I suffered the stigma and I realized the stigma was a result of misinformation.

"People talked about HIV/AIDS, for example, as

being a disease of the promiscuous only. People with wayward behaviors were being punished by God, infected with HIV/AIDS. That was the norm of the thinking among the population." He coughed. "I certainly had relationships with many women before I got married to my wife—I wouldn't call myself a saint in that respect. I was not the promiscuous type, running after everything in skirts—one fling in a year or something like that. But I wouldn't say I was a virgin before I married my wife. It wasn't like that."

He then told me that he was introduced to his first wife in 1990 by a good friend, a trader who had a shop a few streets down from his house. To visit his friend, he would have to pass his future wife selling akara (deep-fried bean-curd balls) on the street in front of her own house. I could see him, younger then, after work sauntering down the dusty road in his black policeman's uniform with its bright red chevrons and short sleeves. I could see her, too—a young face framed by her headscarf, her hands moving skillfully to package the crisp golden snacks for her customers. I could hear the pleasantries exchanged between them as he passed, sure to slow his walk and linger a moment by her stand, alongside the clusters of customers holding money at the ready in one hand and turning up expectant palms in the other.

"I would buy akara from her before proceeding

to where my friend was staying," he said. "That is where myself and the woman developed an interest in each other."

"What about her interested you? What made you fall in love with her?" I asked.

"She was quiet, and I love that," he said, smiling slowly. "She appeared to be somebody who was reserved. She wasn't the noisy type. She wasn't the garrulous type. She didn't want to draw attention to herself. She was somebody who understood me very well. If I was in a bad mood, she knew the mood—I didn't need to tell her—and she could pacify me, change my moods from bad ones to good ones by the understanding and the love that she showed to me. That was what made me to love her."

After a moment, he smiled again and added, "Another thing that made me marry my wife was that she refused to accept my advances. She was different from the other women who were so easy. Certainly, when you're courting a woman in the north, it's improper to enter a sexual relationship with her until you marry her. Any woman from a good family will not allow it, even if you, the man, certainly want."

He paused and then added as an aside, "We as men will demand that."

"But a woman from a good family wouldn't accept that," he continued, "because she thinks that if you have sex with her, you're going to vamoose. That's the normal thing. And yes, I was impatient to see her in my house. We courted for just about six months. Quite short! My friends were actually surprised that I had started falling in love, because at that time, I didn't want things like marriage or women. Honestly, I had already passed the marriageable age. People wanted to see what kind of woman had been able to get me to that stage."

He certainly was a bit older, just over forty when first married—quite unusual for northern Nigeria, where people are often married younger, in their early or midtwenties.

"I was regretting not marrying earlier, because life as a married man was more ordered for me. Certain things I didn't discover single, I discovered them when I was married—some sense of responsibility, a certain sense of being able to save, of being able to lay down some things for a rainy day. I knew that I was now responsible for another person's life. It changed me a lot," he said, nodding deliberately before bringing his palms together and locking his thumbs. We were both quiet as we watched the evening steal across the fields beyond the hospital wall. The sun hovered just above the horizon far out to the west where the town ended abruptly against a mixture of farmland and scrub brush. The women lounging against the building had departed, leaving a scattering of peanut shells now being considered by a band of free-range chickens. "But I'll also tell you that I married again in 1994."

A surprised look must have crossed my face.

"Yes." He continued, either unaware of or unconcerned by my reaction. "While I was with my wife, I married another woman."

He explained that while with the police, he had been transferred from his hometown to the neighboring state as an undercover investigative officer.

"The police station where I worked was close to her house," he said. "She always passed through the police station. I think she was going to her father's house. I was working in the crime department, sitting by the window all the time, and I had the opportunity of seeing her. She caught my eye because of her beauty, very dark skinned and black, and very beautiful—very pretty woman. I one day decided to call upon her. One thing led to another—certainly when I first called her, it was not because of marriage—but one thing led to another and then I married her. I was told her husband had died, but I still married her."

"Was your first wife at all hurt by that?" I asked.

He responded to my question almost before I asked it—as if expecting it.

"Polygamy is not something strange to the two of them," he said. "It's normal. My first wife, she grew up in a polygamous family. Her father had three wives. Certainly no woman wants a rival, however much the culture allows, but it is accepted and my first wife accepted it in good faith. She was also sure that the bond between us was so strong that no other woman could take her place. And it was like that. My first and second wives accepted each other because it had to be like that. I also had a part to play by not showing preference to one or the other. Certainly within the heart of my hearts, the depth of my hearts, my first was the preferred wife, but it was never showed openly, because anything like that will bring conflict." He fell silent. "I was with my second wife for six months, getting to a year, and she started falling sick," Samaila said after his long pause. "And she died. She hadn't got a child for me. We hadn't been pregnant. We hadn't even lived together for too long.

"In the year 2001, my first wife fell very, very sick and was admitted in the hospital. Very luckily for me, the doctor in the hospital was a personal friend. We met most of the time at social gatherings. After my wife had spent three days in the hospital not getting any better, he told me, 'Samaila, let us look for HIV. Let us do an HIV test on your wife.'

"I said, 'No. HIV is for other people. It is not for me. I do not believe that I am infected or that my wife is infected.' He didn't say anything that day, but the next day, he called me again and said, 'Look, Samaila, HIV can come from anything. It can come from a blood donation. It can come from a blood transfusion. It can come from anything. So please, do your best and let us do a test. It is not the end of life.'

"I do remember very well the test was done on a Sunday afternoon around two o'clock. It happened at Yauri at a private hospital, a run-down, ramshackle place. I remember a long bench with hospital equipment on it, and testing vials and needles improperly discarded. It wasn't very neat. I remember the man who did the test at the laboratory was very short, very broad. He told the doctor. The doctor was shivering and washing his hands very fast. I knew something was wrong. He now told me, 'This is what is happening. She is positive.'

"My wife died soon after. I loved her very dearly until the day that she died."

He would later find out that his second wife's first husband had died of HIV/AIDS.

The story Samaila tells of his experience with polygamy and HIV/AIDS does not fit with the polygamy-equals-promiscuity paradigm. It is not the story of a sex-crazed maniac, the societal convention that allows him the ability to fulfill his boundless desires, and the disease that has come to expose how morally backward he is. Rather, it is the experience of a decent and honorable family man struggling to understand how this disease entered into his life. This is not to offer a full-throated defense of polygamy, a practice that sparks debate about the roles and rights of women in a given community; rather, it is to say that within the context of the HIV/AIDS epidemic, one must be careful not to offer simplistic and moralizing conclusions about sexual relationships that exist outside of a certain familiar cultural context. The associated judgment only increases anxiety about the propriety of sexual practice and prevents valuable discussion that might increase understanding of the epidemic's progress. As it turns out, there might be something about a polygamous relationship that speaks to a more generalized pattern of sexual interaction in Nigeria (and sub-Saharan Africa) that may indeed affect the spread of the epidemic, but it has nothing to do with an innate African promiscuity.

Back in New York on a summer day so hot as to make even the most authentically Nigerian person wilt, I paid a visit to Helen Epstein, scientist, journalist, and author of a book on AIDS, *The Invisible Cure*. We sat beneath a large umbrella on the stone patio in the backyard of her Harlem row house, an ice-cold pitcher of water perspiring between us, and discussed the various theories of why HIV/AIDS has spread further and faster in sub-Saharan Africa than in other places.

"It's not that Africans are any more promiscuous than Westerners," I remember her saying. "The average number of lifetime partners is about the same. It's that the patterns of sexual interaction are different."

Patterns of sexual interaction matter tremendously in the spread of the disease. In the West, people tend to engage in sequentially monogamous relationships. In other words, each person has one partner at any one time, with very little overlap between relationships. In such arrangements, a sexually transmitted infection like HIV/AIDS can still pass from person to person, but the completion of one relationship and the establishment of another limit the rate at which it moves. In sub-Saharan Africa—Nigeria included—more emphasis has been placed on the idea of concurrent partnerships, sexual relationships that overlap in time. These overlapping relationships can create a sexual network that, as one study argues, "dramatically increases both the size and variability of an epidemic . . . the speed with which the epidemic spreads." Thus it is likely that HIV/AIDS is more widespread in Africa not because Africans are any more promiscuous or weirdly sexual than other people, but as a result of the presence of sexual networks that allow for increased likelihood of exposure to and transmission of the disease.

A polygamous relationship like Samaila's, because it is so visible and culturally sanctioned, provides an easy and potentially judgment-free example of how concurrency accelerates the spread of HIV in a population. But not all relationships in Nigeria are explicitly culturally sanctioned, though they may still be affected by concurrency. While concurrency counters the idea of a more promiscuous African sexuality as being the cause of the epidemic, it does little to quell the anxiety about the moral quality of sexual relationships that are unsanctioned in this time of HIV/AIDS. These changing relationships are the subject of much agonizing in countries like Nigeria, where increasing urbanization and migration have weakened community control of sexual practice and inspired new ideas about the proper place of sex.

"I know that people are beginning to embrace sex as a human behavior between two adults that you cannot avoid," a young banker I know named Fatimah said to me during one of our many conversations. Her unconscious use of the word *avoid* perfectly expressed the tension that surrounds emerging attitudes toward sex in Nigeria. Many people I spoke with suggested that the proper behavior was waiting until marriage, a comment followed by the caveat "but body no be wood!"—in other words, humans are not inanimate objects and desire eventually wins.

Fatimah always looked every bit the modern African woman. She always dressed very stylishly, multicolored scarves wrapped around her head, wearing thick black-rimmed glasses and crisp black pantsuits with pinstripes or form-fitting dresses cut from traditional fabric.

"Before, if you'd seen two people kissing, it would be a jawbreaker," she said. "It was something that you shouldn't do. People would go, 'Oh my god!' But now it's normal—kissing in public is nothing. People having sex with different partners is a very common thing. I have my circle of friends, and I know how we behave, and I know how we talk. For some people, it's actually very cool for them to talk about having different kinds of partners. I'm sorry to say it, but over here, all the guys, like ninety percent of the guys I know, go casual with sex. They have many partners. It's something that is common. It's something that is normal here. I don't know about the rest of the world, but in Nigeria, a guy having more than one partner is something that is OK."

The official national health survey reports that 26 percent of Nigerian men in both rural and urban areas report having multiple or concurrent partnerships. That is not an insignificant segment of the population and does suggest that concurrency may indeed have cultural roots. I suspect the percentage might actually be higher, given people's tendency to underreport their sexual activity when asked. In fact, some studies have found that when the populations are sorted by age and gender, the number of men in concurrent partnerships rises to 77 percent.

"What about for women?" I asked.

"For here, a girl should not have more than one partner whether married or not," she said. "But now I've noticed the trend is changing. It's becoming more common. It's only normal for a human being to want to have sex, and if you're not getting it with your man and you find yourself in a vulnerable position, you'll end up doing it."

Only 2 percent of Nigerian females report having multiple partners, which reflects the fact that Nigeria is still quite a conservative country when it comes to female sexual behavior. Unfortunately—as is the case in most of the rest of the world—a woman who does not conform to the societal ideal of proper female behavior is quickly and negatively labeled. Thus this statistic is somewhat misleading, for it captures only women who actively seek multiple partners. In reality, many women involved with men who are in multiple partnerships are also in concurrent relationships. Therefore it is probably safe to say that the percentage of women in concurrent relationships— even if not by choice; for example, to avoid extreme poverty—may be close to the percentage of men.

"I've had multiple—if you would call two multiple—partners. That's the most I've had," she continued. "I was single, and then my ex-boyfriend decided to come back. He was like, 'OK. I'm back. I'm serious now. I've got my life straight. Let's do this. Let's get married.' I was there because I thought this guy was serious about me and I don't have any-one, so why not? Let me give it a try and see what will come out of it. And I actually liked him be-fore, so I thought, OK, maybe I'll feel something for him. The other guy—it was just a very rare thing. I met him and we started talking, chatting, meeting. We became very close. We're still very close. So one thing led to another and we had sex and we just liked it. We just enjoyed it. But then the guy is from Imo State, and he's obviously a Christian. He could not take me home, and I could not take him home. It could not happen. His parents are very strong Catho-lics. My parents are Muslims. I'm Hausa. He's Igbo. He's from the south. I'm from the north. We knew it was not going to go anywhere, but we really liked each other. We enjoyed sex. We enjoyed talking. We were good friends."

Fatimah's views reflect a newer, more cosmopolitan philosophy of sexual interaction in which, according to Paulina Makinwa-Adebusoye and Richmond Tiemoko, in their introduction to the book *Human Sexuality in Africa*, " 'shared pleasure' has gained prominence over 'life creation' as amply demonstrated by worldwide declines in fertility and a growing youth culture." HIV/AIDS plays a complicated role in understandings of this new and emerging sexual behavior. On one hand, for those in Nigeria who believe such new attitudes to be wrong, the prevalence of HIV/AIDS demonstrates a pervasive social corruption and thus necessitates a return to traditional ways of sanctioned sexual interaction as delineated by religion or local cultures. For the more progressive, HIV/AIDS has made clear to Nigerians that a world in which everyone waits until marriage to have sex, and once married, has sex only with his or her spouse, is fantasy. It has forced a discussion that reveals we are all having more of the "wrong kind" of sex than we would have initially wanted to admit and therefore are all more exposed to the virus. At the same time, it requires that we modify our notions of sexual morality. The newer HIV/AIDS awareness programs acknowledge this much. No longer can people legitimately preach that we should simply return to abstaining from sex, as our religious

deities and cultural norms demand, in order to prevent the spread of HIV/AIDS, because it is becoming more apparent that such abstinence never really
existed. To do so would be to deny the evidence and
the truism that "body no be wood." In a nod to the
fact that many people are clearly having sex, we now
have public health recommendations like the ABCs
of Sex, first pioneered in Uganda: Abstain, Be mutu-
ally faithful to one partner, and use Condoms if you
can't do the first two. The last directive represents a
monumental shift in the way we in Nigeria, with all
of our religious predilections, think. Though there is
still a cultural norm that condemns all sex outside of
marriage, traditional sexual mores now have to share
the space and in some cases do battle with condoms,
which can be seen as defining a new threshold between legitimate and illegitimate sex. Good sex involves condoms, and bad sex, the kind that spreads
HIV/AIDS, does not.

"Do you use condoms?" I asked Fatimah.

"I practice safe sex. Inasmuch as I want to have
sex and enjoy it, I really, really try so hard to practice
safe sex, 'cause I've seen someone die of HIV, and it's
not a good experience for my family, for her family,
and obviously for the way that she died. I wouldn't
want to put anyone through that. Pregnancy is not
something that I'm scared of, because there are many

ways to get rid of a pregnancy. But there is no way to get rid of AIDS when you get it. I can be pregnant and my parents might be mad at me, but my parents will forgive me. God will forgive me, and I will live to raise my child. But if I have HIV, I will be hurting my parents, because people begin to judge you, and that's what I don't want. I would rather not have that shame and painful death in the future. I would just rather use the protection."

It is telling that at one point in our conversation, Fatimah told me, "Even if my husband ends up sleeping around, I've already prepared my mind on how to control it. I don't want a husband who sleeps around without protection. I'm the type that would pack my husband's traveling case with condoms inside. I was telling my boyfriend that if he has to cheat on me—and he was like 'No! No! No! Stop telling me this. You're trying to put ideas in my head!'—I was like, 'No! If you have it in you, you will do it. I'm just giving you my own little conditions. *Please, please, please*, safe sex whatever you do. And don't bring it near me.' I'd rather handle the situation at hand. I'd rather tell him these are my conditions if you have to do it. 'Cause I know, sometimes we're all human."

A majority of Nigerians know about condoms, even if we do not always use them correctly or consistently. Ninety percent of people in urban areas and

64 percent of people in rural areas have heard of male condoms. You can find them in hotels and gas stations, in drugstores and even roadside kiosks. Nigerians have used over 900 million condoms since 2002, and that number will only rise. They are here to stay, and they are changing the way we have sex, but the relationship we have with them is complex.

"For example," a driver I know named Obong told me as we sat at a brukutu joint where he had taken me for an after-work chat, "now, if I see you with a girl, I will now tell you, 'Remember your bulletproof.' I will now tell you, 'If you see a big river—like river Niger or Benue—instead of you to sleep with this girl without condom, so it is better for you to use block, put rope on it, hang it on your neck, and jump inside river.'" He wrapped an invisible rope around his neck and then pantomimed tossing a heavy cinder block over the edge into a river, followed, after a short pause, by his body.

Obong returned to our coarse wooden bench beneath a flamboyant tree with its red blossoms and fanned himself slowly with that morning's folded newspaper. His shirt bore dark sweat stains where it folded into the creases of his body. He was not an especially large man, but he joked about his growing potbelly and how the extra weight made him sweat a little harder. Around us sprawled a chaotic convention of bars and brothels connected to illegally rigged extensions from the power grid. Men sat in groups, holding bottles of Guinness stout or Star beer as they conversed loudly with one another. Ignored and unhindered, roaming goats gnawed the sackcloth walls of temporary buildings and nuzzled the ground for bits of rubbish.

"To commit suicide is better than you to go on that girl without condom," he said again. "Because you should remember what is happening in the town. If you should go enter like that, it means you use rope, tie your neck like that, jump in river. From that you understand where you're going."

His dramatic endorsement of condoms reflects a sentiment that is remarkably widespread in Nigeria. However, while awareness about condoms and their role in stopping the spread of HIV/AIDS is high, condom usage is despairingly low. Only 28 percent of sexually active Nigerians have ever used a condom during intercourse and, as expected, there is more condom use in urban areas than in rural areas. The question, of course, is why—if people know about condoms and their role in preventing HIV/AIDS, why are they not using them?

There are a number of possible reasons why people don't use condoms during sexual intercourse, many of which point to the anxiety generated by the sexual experience. First, both men and women the world over agree that sex feels better without condoms. A number of studies suggest that this is the number one reason why people do not use condoms when having sex. This is probably as true in the United States as it is in Nigeria and throughout Africa. Furthermore, condoms can be expensive for the average person in Nigeria, who hasn't much disposable income. Condoms are also awkward. They are awkward to buy, even in the passionately liberal New York City, as they make a bold statement about one's sexual activities. This may be more true in Nigeria, where sex is not discussed as openly as in other places. A number of people I spoke with said shopkeepers cast disapproving glances in their direction when they tried to buy condoms. Some received sermons about the sinful nature of premarital sex. Worse, some women were propositioned immediately upon leaving the store. Condoms also break the flow of romance and passion. One young man told me that he thought guys don't like to use condoms because putting one on gives both parties the chance to consider how sinful sex is. Another young man told me about a university friend who avoided that awkward moment, when the girl might say no while he was putting on the condom, by donning one before going out for the night. Then there are the rumors, the most pervasive and destructive of which is that condoms often break.

"That's just it," Obong said when I asked him what he thought about the idea that condoms are unreliable. He then elaborated. "I was on this assignment in the south, and there was this girl. She was just making phone call when I passed. She was in a wheelchair," he continued. "All this wheelchair that First Lady used to dash people that cannot walk.* That's the wheelchair she were using, rolling it with her hand. If you see her, how she fat and sit on the wheelchair, you think maybe she look like somebody who has a baby at hand. She's a pretty girl even though she's paralyzed—keep herself very neat, with long hair. Since she sit down in the wheelchair, I believe that people doesn't rush to her like these other beautiful ones that pass. See, when you see a beautiful girl, it's not only you that see her; many people see her, but those who have money, they go on her. I was not with enough money to spend for all those kind big girls in that area. I now look at her in that way that if I succeed, it will not cost me a lot. Since she agree, I now come to her place later in the evening, since I have that appointment with her. And I just buy her little provision, buy her something in

---

* Refers to a program for the disabled championed by Nigeria's then first lady Turai Yar'Adua.

the leather," he said, referring to plastic grocery bags that, for reasons I have never understood, Nigerians call leather.

"So what happened?" I asked.

"Well, I play with her. I was trying to touch her breasts, play—you know, in romantic way—for her to make a move so that she can allow me to do my aim of coming there. She enjoy me. And I fire her very well. Then I now realize that the taste of my coming to release was now not like when I start. I think you understand?"

I nodded. The condom was no longer in place.

"You know by that time you reach, at the point of release, it has no control at that time. Even if they point you gun, you think, you feel, let them shoot. But it's only till when you come down from there you now realize that 'Ah! So somebody is standing here with gun to shoot me!' So I keep on till when I release. After I release, I now find out that the rope of the neck of the condom was on my prick. I now find out that the condom tear. I now ask her to check where is the remaining condom. I even put hand in her private part to look for it—whether the thing cut and go inside. Nothing. The condom tear and now fold as I'm seriously injecting. I now find that all my sperm has released inside her private part. I say, 'Wow!' I say, 'Well, it has happened. It has happened.

Since this thing has happened like this, any STD, surely if she has, I will take it. If it is STD—whether nah HIV or not—if God says I should take it, I will take it. If God says I will not take it, then OK.'" He shivered in remembrance of the moment.

"What did you do after the condom broke?" I asked.

He released a guarded smile and spoke slowly. "After that thing tear, I did not even care to use even the second condom I was having. I say, 'After all, I already release into her.' She let me know I'm fit. I'm a man; I fire her five times. I have to continue. I have to."

What would you do at this moment? What would I do? Almost every sexually active person has experienced a broken condom. It causes an intense anxiety even as it generates a certain rush from exposure to the risk of pregnancy or disease. In my friend's case, his feelings illustrate the larger dilemma and complexity of choices that people face in a time of changing moral standards and attitudes about sex. The belief that sex outside of marriage is wrong still holds sway even as we acknowledge that in practice we often ignore moral convention. Condoms are often seen as tools that enable sin or wrongdoing even if they do provide the benefit of protection against HIV/AIDS. But condoms also diminish sexual pleasure and are considered faulty. They raise the question: if certain kinds of sex are sinful and possible punishment in the form of HIV/AIDS awaits anyway, why mitigate the pleasure of the sin? Many people make that decision and forgo condoms despite the risks. For others the result is mental and emotional gymnastics that seek to take the sin out of sex and in so doing remove the threat of HIV as a possible consequence or punishment. The anthropologist Daniel Jordan Smith describes one of the main ways this is done in Nigeria as moral partnering, the construction of sexual relationships in the language of monogamy and religion, in which relationship morality is associated with decreased risk of exposure to HIV/AIDS.

On one of my trips to Lagos, in 2007, I had a long chat with Dele, a university student who explained the idea very clearly: "So basically me, I believe that if you love somebody—as in when, I mean, you *love* somebody, you have to be faithful to the person for you to even love the person. I'm using myself now as an example. My ex-girlfriend—I was faithful to her to the core. I trusted her. I still trust her, you get? If you and your partner trust each other, I don't think there's going to be any room for fear of AIDS or any kind of sexual disease."

He spoke loudly, but it was hard to hear him over the din outside. We sat by a lectern in a chapel in the compound of a mutual acquaintance. A carved wooden Jesus looked down at us from a simple wooden altar. It was election season then, and the politicking was in full swing. Along the streets, political posters covered nearly every available surface, and vans laden with speakers blasting the advertising jingles of the various candidates could be heard even inside. Dele was a physics major at the well-regarded University of Lagos. Freshly barbered with his hair brushed forward and smoothed to a black shine with sweet-smelling oil, wearing a pressed short-sleeve shirt, stylish jeans, and sneakers that were impossibly white, given the dusty streets outside, he looked more like a GQ model than a physics nerd. He made me incredibly self-conscious of my rumpled green tie-dyed shirt and hair that I hadn't had cut in months.

"Tell me about your girlfriend," I said.

"She's my ex-girlfriend now," he said, shifting his weight in an uncomfortable orange plastic chair. "She's the girl I'm still going to get married to, because I pray to God about it. I used to be seriously crazy about the girl. I'm still crazy about her. She was a very beautiful, reserved girl. She's pretty." His hands clutched each other, massaged each other as he sat otherwise still, causing a flutter in his sleeves. "Yeah. She has very good shape, very lovely shape. Yeah. Fit," he said. "She was a virgin." He made sure to point this out. "I just wanted to date her. I don't know *sha*. Probably I just wanted to sleep with her or something when I first met her. She was really proving stubborn and everything. OK, I now started liking her *sha*. Then we started dating. She's the best thing. She changed my life. Seriously, she changed my life. I started breaking up with a lot of girls. I broke up with like half of my girlfriends in the first two weeks."

"Sorry," I interrupted. "You said you broke up with half of your girlfriends?"

"Then, officially, I had eight girlfriends," he said with a smile. "I didn't have time again for girls like that. As in she had this one kind of impact on me. Then later, after about one month or so, I broke up with everybody apart from one other girl. I really liked that girl too. Then along the line, after one and a half years, I just had to choose one."

How can you be faithful to more than one person? I didn't understand it at first, but Dele's story shows the mental and emotional constructs people create to cope with prohibitions against sex. In the realm of moral partnering, the terms *boyfriend* and *girlfriend* have positive moral connotations and are thus preferably used to describe relationships. A person can potentially have more than one moral partner at a time, as the start of one relationship might overlap with the end of another. Condom usage is not high in these relationships because it suggests the possibility of "one's own or one's partners' infidelity." Furthermore, I imagine that asking whether or not a partner has been tested for HIV would also imply that the person is or has been immoral. These factors lead to a mental picture of low risk of exposure to HIV that does not translate into reality.

The reality of the situation is that we all, when we make the decision to be sexually active, place ourselves at some risk of exposure to HIV/AIDS. While some groups may be more at risk than others, the virus has the potential to infect all sexually active people. This should not be a cause for alarm and further restrictive grouping or meaningless prohibition of sexual activity. Rather, it should lead us to more open and accepting discussion about what Samaila, the former police officer, called "the greatest pleasures of life: love, sex." By understanding how sex in Nigeria—indeed, throughout Africa and the world—influences and is influenced by the presence of HIV/AIDS, we can better enable ourselves to halt the epidemic's progress.

DEATH

On one of my trips to Nigeria, Doc and Samaila introduced me to a man named Ikenna, who ran a bar on the same military base where I happened to meet Elizabeth. He was small, with short arms protruding from the rolled sleeves of a blue, orange, and green dashiki. The fabric engulfed him so completely that his body wandered within it even as he sat perched on the edge of his plastic seat. I wiped my forehead and face repeatedly with a paper napkin that dissolved into bits that stuck to my sideburns and beard. He didn't sweat, not a drop or even a shine on his forehead in the low lights as he sat across from me. He was extremely attentive, carefully monitoring and measuring the proximity of opportunity (a customer) or the velocity of danger (a drunk customer). He kept a steady watch over his bar girls, ready to berate them into skips and smiles as they suffered the indignities of heat, the buckets heavy with bottles of drink they carried, and the catcalls of intoxicated men. His eyes were pulled down into a tired, wary slant by a persistent frown. He had a potbelly that was visible when he stood momentarily to see what business, if any, needed attending to while we spoke.

That night, clouds intermittently obscured the moon, and in the low light, I watched soldiers milling about; even though drunk, they carefully avoided old divots filled with a collected mess of wash water and carelessly discarded drink. They shouted hearty greetings in the local Hausa language, "Sanu! Sanu!" or pidgin English, "How now!" with handshakes pulled into hugs, then released again into handshakes that ended in snaps. Colored lights played across the open courtyard and bounced to the rhythm of the music blasting through the loudspeakers: 2Face Idibia's "African Queen"—"You are my African queen, the girl of my dreams"—was the popular song of the moment, and it seemed to play on repeat. Between the beer and Coke bottles, over the wood-smoked suya, peppered meat, which Ikenna and I jealously protected from persistent flies, we tossed some conversation starters back and forth—"Did you see the Super Eagles play? Why can't our boys just play good football anymore?"—the neutral subjects you speak of when you know a person only so well and talk centers on common subjects: rainy season versus dry season, country calm versus city chaos.

"You're welcome," Ikenna said to me softly, without warmth, after the chitchat dissipated. I put my notebook on the table between us and he watched with interest as I leafed through to a blank page.

"So," I said, bouncing my knees, "tell me about yourself."

He settled into his seat for a moment, slid his traditional cap off his head into his lap, revealing a closely shaved head, hairline receded into a deep W, and sighed.

Ikenna was much older than he looked. Originally from the east, he was the son of a poor farmer. He was supposed to go to college, to lift his family from poverty with his education and perhaps a career in the civil service, business, or medicine, but his terrible exam results at the end of secondary school prevented that. Instead he got on a bus with his few possessions in a bag, his only guide the address of an older sister who had married a man from Kontangora, a small town near the military base, and began the journey north. His first job was managing bars, then he moved into brothels, and then after Sharia law became a problem for certain establishments, he moved into selling drinks on a military base. Twenty years later, he was still here, but at some point along the way, he had gotten HIV.

Every so often, Ikenna cocked his head to one side to better watch his serving girls walk to and from his stall. They stepped into the orange light and in one swift motion deftly swept one arm to their breasts to keep cleavage in place while quickly swapping empty beer bottles for cold full ones. Mist from the deep freezer where the drinks were stored engulfed them. Ikenna, it seems, was not a man who trusted easily.

"Can we talk about HIV?" I asked after a long pause.

"You're welcome," he said again.

Here? Now? In the open, where everyone's conversation was common property and someone might overhear our discussion? I had whispered the word *HIV*, as people do when speaking the uncomfortable.

He read my face. It was late. He had to work. Maybe we could get together after his HIV/AIDS support-group meeting. He presented all of this calmly, as life's simple and obvious routine.

I took his number.

"Can I come to the meeting?" I asked, my words faltering, almost dissipating in the distance between us.

He responded with a light shove of the table as he pushed his chair back and stood. The bottles lined up on its surface rattled. "Why not?"

The support group met at the local hospital, where large orange-tailed lizards scurried across courtyards of struggling crabgrass bobbing their heads at one another, tasting the air with their tongues. The Hausa men who worked as nurses wore white safari suits as uniforms. They slipped in and out of the wards and headed for the afternoon prayers toward a small mosque built on the hospital grounds. The support group's meeting room was on one side of the hospital, near the recovery ward for men who had just had hernias repaired. They met in a small cube of a room with cracked plaster and a small window high in one wall that allowed a thin sheet of sunlight to catch dust particles stirred by a wobbling ceiling fan.

When all members had assembled, they mulled over a list of concerns and joys no different from those of average Nigerians: "I have no food for my family." "I need school fees for my children." "Money for housing." "A job." "My boy just finished his West African Examination Council exam." "My sister needs to do a traditional wedding." Then someone said, "My drugs have failed." There was an audible gasp. Nobody said a word. The women tugged at their headscarves.

The voice belonged to a young man in a muscle shirt that showed off defined biceps and prominent veins. Someone put a hand on his back, rubbed, and mumbled, "It will be OK. What line of medication?"

"Second line. Kaletra," the man said, taking his time so as to control an aggravated stutter.

"You don't have to worry too much," his comforter said, and then loudly for everyone else to hear, to relieve tension, ease away collective fear. "There is still third line, and in some cases you can even go back to first line. It will be OK."

A heaviness had settled upon the room. I watched as Ikenna slipped outside. I followed.

"Can we talk?" I asked, finally relieved to have him alone and in a quiet space.

He nodded. "You want me to tell you what I know about the something?" Ikenna rasped. "In fact I never knew about the something the first time I was very seriously feeling sick. They took me to hospital. I got OK," he continued as we walked away from the hospital buildings down a path trampled through the grass toward a road that looped around the hospital grounds. Gravel crunched beneath our sandals as we approached hazy shapes of bungalows set back from the road on long drives. "Within some weeks, it started again, and they say I should go for a test. They say it's HIV. I say, 'No, it can't be. I have not been meddling with women for a long time.' So I resisted. I say, 'No! I have to move to Kaduna to do another test.' When I got there, to one big military hospital, they tested me, and it's the same thing. Since that time, I accepted it. It was the year 2000."

As we walked on, chatting, I noticed that he had trouble breathing and would pull his air in sharply, in between the bits and pieces he told me about his life. I asked him a number of times if he wanted to stop, but he waved away my concern with a small hand. At one point, as the road looped back toward the hospital compound, taking us from the hot sun into the shade of large trees planted in perfect lines, I turned to him and asked, "Ikenna. Do you ever wish you didn't have HIV?"

He answered very quickly. "No." There was no equivocation in his voice, not even a hint of lamentation about the things that he might never know or see—his three children growing up and marrying. There was no hint of a fear of death.

"Tot! Nah God gets us? Once they tell you, you have to accept. It is their job. So they told me. I have to accept," he said as we entered the hospital through the men's hernia recovery ward. Around us, patients shifted in their beds, groaning, mumbling prayers, and straining against painful coughs. We moved quickly and quietly so as not to disturb them. "I thank God I'm still getting up to eat," he whispered to me. "I feel fine, so I have no fear over it. There are some—you see the way they appear—you know that thing is worrying them. When it enters into them too much, it used to destroy body. You see some lean, looking like a broom. I thank God I'm not looking like them."

We pledged to continue our conversation the next

time I came to Kontangora. I didn't know that that would be the first and last time I spoke with him. Two months later, as I sat at John F. Kennedy Airport in New York waiting to board a British Airways flight back to Nigeria, I received a short e-mail from Samaila.

"Your friend Ikenna is dead," he wrote. "He died last week of a respiratory infection."

I sat there staring out the window at the large body of the plane I was about to board, stunned. A living, breathing someone who was once here was now not. The connection that we had started to form—suddenly cut short. I stood there, mouth open, eyes wide, fully aware of the breath flowing in and then out of me, paralyzed by a profound sense of the incomplete, another death caused by HIV/AIDS.

From the moment of its first presentation, HIV/ AIDS has been intimately associated with death, and necessarily so. The first cases to appear in the United States were those people with advanced HIV infections, end-stage AIDS. No one knew the exact cause, but the effect was clear; without exception, these people died. Even after HIV was isolated as the cause of the constellation of symptoms that consti- tute AIDS, there were no effective drugs or vaccines to treat the virus, and people still died. Only in the mid-1990s, after the introduction of powerful antiviral drug cocktails and massive public education programs, did death as a result of HIV/AIDS become less immediate. Though the scope of the sub-Saharan African HIV/AIDS epidemic became clear after the introduction of lifesaving treatments in the West, this epidemic has followed a similar trajectory. An initial lack of access to treatment meant that the majority of people who contracted HIV/AIDS in sub-Saharan Africa would die. In recent years, as public health programs have become more effective in their outreach and access to treatment increases throughout the continent, things are changing. Still, first impressions are hard to shake. Over twenty years and many medical advancements later, people still believe, as one young man I met said, "What I know about the HIV problem is that HIV don't have cure in life. If you have HIV, your world is gone. If you have something calling HIV, know that you will lose your life."

When considering the sub-Saharan HIV/AIDS epidemic, many find it difficult not to adopt this attitude. The numbers alone make it hard to believe that this disease brings anything but death. In 2009, 1.3 million people in sub-Saharan Africa died from HIV/AIDS. In Nigeria there were over two hundred thousand AIDS-related deaths that same year. But what does this all mean?

Development indicators have traditionally been one of the ways that we interpret the impact of mass casualties in this epidemic, and the impact is deep. To begin with, it's not just that people die; it's who dies that makes HIV/AIDS so powerful. Most diseases tend to cause death among the very old or the very young, but this epidemic is most deadly among the sexually active, those between the ages of fifteen and fifty, who also make up the majority of any given country's working population. As a result, the mortality rate in a given population is increased when it should be at its lowest.

In addition, because the epidemic affects women more than men, a traditional pattern in mortality is changing. Normally the death rate among women is lower than among men, but with HIV/AIDS, women are dying at earlier ages and in greater numbers, because women are biologically and socially more vulnerable to HIV.

Finally, life expectancy has decreased as a result of the epidemic. The average life expectancy for a person from sub-Saharan Africa is now fourteen years less than it would be had HIV/AIDS never existed, dropping a life expectancy already much lower than in the rest of the world down to an astoundingly brief forty-five years. This loss of life exacts an economic cost, further exacerbating what I have heard some people in Nigeria jokingly call AIDS—African Inability-to-Develop Syndrome. Countries affected by HIV/AIDS deaths face a declining workforce, which can translate into a drastic drop in productive capacity. Household incomes drop dramatically when working members of a family die from HIV/AIDS. Most alarmingly, when adults die from HIV/AIDS, they leave behind children, orphans, who will likely have decreased access to nutrition, educational opportunities, and other economic advantages that would make them productive members of society. In general, the standard of living decreases and whole societies fall further behind. Death from HIV/AIDS comes to mean a loss of opportunity, not just for those who die, but for those they leave behind.

We often prefer these statistical interpretations and macroeconomic analyses of HIV/AIDS-related death, primarily because the numbers seem more tangible. Decreased economic output, reduced GDP, and a household that now lacks income are easily represented as the consequence of this epidemic. But I also wonder whether a focus on economic deprivation when considering HIV/AIDS-related death in Africa is ultimately reductive, casting Africans as an amalgam of physical needs and in the process overlooking the real sense of missing another person that humanizes the experience.

When I spoke with Fatimah, the banker, about her aunt who had died of HIV/AIDS, she said of her family's experience, "Whenever we're together, we can all feel her loss in the air. It's there." As she spoke, her voice softened until it was almost inaudible and her face relaxed into the contours of sadness.

"When it started she used to smoke, so she thought she had tuberculosis. The doctors told her she had tuberculosis. Finally after two years, she went to a hospital in Kano. They tested her and they told her she had HIV. Obviously they didn't deliver the message well. You know Nigerian doctors, they just come out and say you have HIV. They don't go through counseling and talking to you, making you understand this is something you can live with. They just tell you, 'OK, you have HIV.' She broke down. Everything happened in the span of two months. She took herself to the hospital, but she didn't come out walking. They had to carry her out of the hospital and she was on bed rest—sick. Two months after, she passed.

"I was very close to her. She was actually my mom's cousin, but they grew up together. Everything, they did together. I grew up with my cousin who was her daughter. We were just like one family. She was a mother to me. I didn't see her as an aunt. I could go to her for anything. So losing her was . . . that was my first major loss.

"What was she like—your aunt?" I asked her.

"She was tall, really tall, like six one, and she

had this beautiful shape, long hair, pretty smile, caramel skin. She was a great person. She laughed a lot. She was always laughing, and she laughed out loud. She was a storyteller. She was a mother. She had all the qualities of a mother, and she was nice to everyone, kind and giving."

Fatimah stopped speaking for a moment and drew in a deep breath.

"I still miss her. I do. And when I see my cousin, I can see the tension. I think partly I'm over it; I'm able to deal with it now. I think her daughter is even stronger than I am when it comes to discussing her and her past."

Fatimah's experience with her aunt's death reminds us that death is an individual emotional experience. Numbers alone do not make death meaningful. Rather, they create a spectacle that captures attention for a moment before alienating its beholder in a realm of fact. That a young woman must sit and consider all the emotions that arise in a life without her aunt makes us question how we would behave in the same situation and so deepens our understanding of her humanity.

This small globe of a virus with its sinister round spikes is by now a familiar picture for many people in the world. It has been a celebrity of sorts, even receiving its own magazine covers and spreads. So intense is this association of HIV/AIDS and death that the diagnosis of HIV is itself considered the end of life. As the former police officer and activist, Samaila, explained to me, "Immediately I realized I was HIV positive, certainly what came over my mind at that time is that I was going to die. I knew—or I thought—I was about to die, and I was sure of that. So the first thing I did was that I put in a retirement letter, a resignation letter, from the police force so that I would be able to take any gratuities that were due to me, build a house for my children, and then go ahead and die. It was as fatal as that."

Even more devastating is the fact that the HIV-positive person loses his or her identity to the virus, becoming a form of death incarnate. The living human body becomes a visible reminder of the same decay that happens to a corpse. In the words of a man who described a woman he knew who died from HIV/AIDS, "How can one woman with hip like this, breast like this—full breast—just turn into nothing? Nothing? Her body change color—a yellow lady become a black. Her whole body just disappear and cover in rashes to the point where you cannot even look at her. You just cannot."

We do not like to look at death. It has remained

abstract primarily because we have separated ourselves from its physical form through ceremony and ritual designed to control or appease the violence it offers. Burial, cremation, and the ceremonies that surround them allow for an effective disposal of death in its physical form while providing a platform for the collective expression of the emotions death calls forth. HIV/AIDS flouts these culturally constructed barriers between the worlds of the living and the dead and in so doing disrupts the normal process of grieving.

Obong, the driver from Abuja, had lost seven friends to HIV/AIDS. He had even driven the coffins of his friends from Abuja to their villages and final resting places. Death from HIV/AIDS was not new to him, nor were the associated burials.

"Like in my place," he said as we sat there, "if somebody die, if they have children, if they bury you, your family will not go to farm until seven days. That is the respect they will give to you because you are family man. Maybe they hear that this other village trespass, find trouble, kill our youth. If you see the kind [of] burial they will give to such person, you will now know that yes, you were a good person in society. When you die, if because of that HIV and AIDS, your burial will just be as if they bury dog. They will say, 'What are they keeping you for? You were not responsible. You did not leave anything behind, no legacy. So there is no need of feel-ing pains.' I'm telling you this. As far as youth just dig hole, they put you there; they cover. The next day, people go to their farm, continue their life. It's just like this bird flu killing fowl. They will say the breeze have touched you, so they have to bury you according to the way you live your life." He sat qui-etly after he finished speaking, and sighed heavily.

It appears that in Nigeria, death comes in fla-vors: good and bad. A good death is one that unites a community in its emotion and allows for public expression of grief. In a good death, the deceased is someone who in life strengthened the fabric of soci-ety by contributing and through death has the power to do the same by bringing people together. The death of an elderly person who leaves behind family and the death of a young person in the service of the community are life affirming. Death in these situa-tions is seen as normal and reflective of good charac-ter. A bad death is one that divides a community and is either indicative of or results from bad character. Because HIV/AIDS confuses the lines between life and death, it turns death into an abnormal, unnatural process. This kind of death cannot be ceremonial-ized. There is no gathering of community, no ex-pression of collective emotion. There is the sense of something incomplete.

"That is how life is," Obong finally said. "There's no two way about it. If you dance good, you dance to the end. But when you dance bad, you dance halfway."

He readjusted his shades to fully cover his eyes with the shimmering blue lenses. He didn't look at me.

The link between HIV/AIDS and death is especially hard to sever, but the way we think about HIV/AIDS and death is changing—primarily because so many people living with HIV/AIDS have fought to reimagine the perceived death the rest of the world assumes they live.

In Lagos, at their offices near a Julius Berger Construction Company staging ground by the lagoon, I met an HIV-positive woman who worked for the Nigerian Business Coalition Against AIDS (NIBUCAA), a foundation set up by a consortium of companies—Julius Berger included—addressing the issue of HIV/AIDS in Nigeria. We spoke just outside the office, so as not to disturb her colleagues working inside. The air smelled of diesel and industrial products, and the landscape that stretched out before us was bleak. Crushed gravel, chain-link fences, scrap metal, rebar, and other building products, along with the constant churning noise of large trucks exiting and entering the premises, gave the setting a postapocalyptic feel. We stood in a corner of a carport freshly painted in white. An odd collection of black butterflies fluttered around a Mercedes parked in front of us.

"Like for me when I just tested, I'm used to wearing trousers and tops—small tops," she said as we leaned against the wall. She had the slight frame of a fashion model, if a little short, with a delicate face framed by her relaxed hair. Her skirt suit was cut to just above her knees, and her smooth calves tapered into a pair of black dress shoes.

"And then all of a sudden I start wearing something long," she continued. "I would cover my head. I won't talk to people. I wanted to stop schooling. When after we knew it was HIV, my strength was very low, and at that stage I wished death could come. There was one day, two days I didn't take my bath, but death didn't come. Death didn't come. Then I decided to take my bath. And despite the fact I used hot water, I was cold. I was shaking. And I prayed to God that if death did not take me now, then I should be able to live and *live*. After that night I was just praying that if death could not take me now, then I'm going to live long. Then one day I just said, It seems you're hiding. Are you ashamed of yourself? Why are you ashamed? You still have a lot to live for. Your father and mother still believes in you. Your family still believes in you. You can still do something. I started my medication December 2004. Then I bounced back to life. I went back to school—although I had an extra semester because I missed all my exams. And I just moved on in life. Ever since then, I've always been on the move. I'm always on the move."

I could believe it. As we talked, she constantly bounced her shoulder against the wall. She seemed so possessed of energy and motion that I wondered how she was able to work at a desk in an office.

"The next question I asked myself was, I have to learn about this disease that wants to kill me. I started going to the Net, go to the Web, start searching for 'human immunodeficiency virus,' the virus I believed would kill me. But eventually you find out more, that this virus does not eventually kill. Other opportunistic infection kills the person. And if the person is at the stage of denial, the person may end up dead. So that's how I became open about my status. I learned more. I started going to workshops, trainings. Another thing I did was to join a support group, AIDS Alliance Nigeria. I remember the first time I went to support group. I saw more than two hundred. People that are older than me. People that are younger than me. I said, 'Ah! So all these people are living with HIV.' The thing that amazed me even was that they were quarreling about they were supposed to give them food. They were quarreling about it—transport allowance. I was like, 'Ah-ah? These people are not even thinking at all about death.' I was just amazed, and that inspired me like, if these people can live and still struggle like this, I can do more things.

"It's not as if I'm really proud to be living with HIV, but I felt there's a need for me to be doing something positively. And the way to affect people's lives positively is to let people know that OK, the message is true—it's a fact. Because a lot of people believe that AIDS is not real. And for me to do that, I have to become open about my status. I have to tell people. And after telling them the message that this person you're seeing is really living with HIV, and she's been coping, and if she can cope, you too can cope. And if she's positive, then anybody can be positive as well. And if you're negative, there are steps you can take to remain negative and live your life as well."

In her essay "Beyond the Politics of Bare Life," the anthropologist Jean Comaroff writes, "Claiming positive identity can be tantamount to a conversion experience: quite literally a path to salvation. . . . Rebirth through the disease likewise involves standardized formulas of self-declaration, a passage to new ontological certainty and transparency that claims to reverse the deceptions of prejudice, secrecy, and un-truth." This is to say that there is life after perceived death, that it can be lived completely, fully, and with renewed purpose, that being positive, in both senses, can engender a new HIV/AIDS paradigm that em-phasizes life. In the words of another activist I spoke with, an Igbo man who had been HIV positive for ten years, "Life begins when you know your status. If you don't know your status, life has never begin. Like that 2001, I know my status, that is a new life I begin. . . . It's a new life."

This new life begins only after an intense reckon-ing with HIV/AIDS-related death. It does not come by ignoring or denying the fact that HIV/AIDS can kill even under the best of circumstances—after all, Ikenna was compliant with his treatments and very active in his community of HIV-positive people—but by recognizing that each individual death is impor-tant, because it represents the loss of a human con-nection. Preserving and enhancing these connections in the face of the epidemic can serve as the motiva-tion for further action.

In recent years, there has been a downward trend in the number of HIV/AIDS-related deaths in sub-Saharan Africa. In Nigeria, the number of reported deaths related to AIDS has stabilized and is no lon-ger increasing. As fewer people die and the number of people living openly, positively, and productively increases, it becomes harder and harder to complete the equation HIV/AIDS equals death. And as these people live fuller, more visible lives, more accepted lives, their presence and vocality demand a discussion not only about what HIV/AIDS means in a community, but also about how that community can ensure that all people, positive or not, are positively influenced by the epidemic.

SPEAKING OF AIDS

Nigerians are not known as a quiet people. "In the beginning," writes the Nigerian essayist Peter Enahoro, "God created the universe; then He created the moon, the stars and the wild beasts of the forests. On the sixth day, He created the Nigerian and there was peace. But on the seventh day while God rested, the Nigerian invented noise." Ours is a noisy country, so loud sometimes that, even in rural areas, it can be difficult to hear your own thoughts above the constant commotion of Nigerian life. At all times, somewhere someone is offering greetings, arguing, partying. The streets of our cities and the dirt roads of our small towns teem with a million conversations held over the background noise of music blasting from car speakers or twanging out from tiny handheld radios, as well as the nearly constant rattle and rumble of ubiquitous standby generators. We are opinionated, and we are loud even when wrong. We protest and we riot. We do not shy away from controversy. And perhaps because we are rooted in an oral culture, we revel in the sounds of our own voices: introductory remarks take up volumes; toasts leave raised arms trembling; speeches, if they ever end, never end before the speaker's time is up. But for all the talking we do, until relatively recently, we have been noticeably silent on the subject of HIV/AIDS.

If the current HIV/AIDS epidemic has a characteristic that sets it apart from other epidemics, it is that this is the only mass outbreak of disease that has happened quietly. In fact, so quietly did it spread that for the first twenty years of the epidemic, as a society we had to question whether HIV/AIDS was actually real. This is changing. Recently there has been more of a collective acknowledgment that HIV/AIDS is very real. It is now a term that everybody knows something about, and this is reshaping the way we behave toward the virus and people who have it. Speaking more openly about the disease, while not a solution to the epidemic in and of itself, is an important first step.

This is a disease that thrives on silence. The virus is a quiet pathogen without any specific disease markers that make it easily differentiable from other illnesses. It usually displays symptoms that announce its presence only at the very end of an infected person's life. Those who have it and those who have recently contracted it don't necessarily know they have it unless they specifically ask. Those who do know they have it are often quiet about their status because of stigma and discrimination.

In Nigeria, the most prominent person to die of HIV/AIDS was the popular Afro-beat musician Fela Kuti, whom I mentioned earlier. Fela was one of the country's most flamboyant entertainers and loudest activists, a perpetual voice of protest and a constant thorn in the side of Nigeria's ruling elite. He often performed his songs of social commentary and protest shirtless, sometimes in nothing more than a pair of skimpy briefs. The author of songs like "Shuffering and Shmiling," which chronicled the indignities of everyday working-class Nigerian life, or "Zombie," which articulated many a Nigerian's disgust with a succession of oppressive military regimes, Fela came as close as possible to representing what one might call the voice of the people in a chaotically pluralistic country like Nigeria. He also lived what has been called a "safe-sex educator's nightmare," swearing off condoms and maintaining a rotating system of twelve wives after initially marrying twenty-seven women in one ceremony. Despite his brother's role as minister of health during the 1980s and the architect of Nigeria's initial response to the HIV/AIDS epidemic, Fela refused to believe that he had the condition, let alone to speak out about its presence and impact on Nigerian life. Some have criticized him for this position, given his stature and great influence. In 1997, he died from Kaposi's sarcoma—an AIDS-related cancer—and through his death probably did more to galvanize a fledgling HIV/AIDS movement in the country than he ever could have while alive. The announcement by his brother, Dr. Olikoye Ransome-Kuti, that Fela had died from AIDS was the first time many Nigerians had ever heard of the disease, despite its long existence in the country.

"When my father was diagnosed with HIV/AIDS, we couldn't understand," Fela's son, the world-renowned Afro-beat star Femi Kuti, said to me when I met him at his New Africa Shrine in Lagos. The shrine was built on a concept similar to his father's earlier Kalakuta Republic. The Shrine, as it is simply and commonly known, is a concert hall with living space and offices in the back, in the heart of the Ikeja section of Lagos. It is open to all regardless of status. More than anything else, the New Africa Shrine resembles a large open-air warehouse with a stage at one end, a bar at the other, and plastic tables and chairs haphazardly arranged on the concrete space in between.

When I spoke with Femi Kuti, the air was heavy with the smell of marijuana and music pulsed from large speakers near the stage. I sat with Femi on a balcony overlooking the scene below. He held a shining brass saxophone in his lap and fingered the keys as he spoke. It was somewhat disconcerting to sit across from him because he bears an uncanny resemblance to his father: the same high cheekbones, skeptical eyes, and semipermanent frown.

"We didn't understand what they were talking about," he said. He was surprisingly soft-spoken for a man with such a large stage presence. "His case was the first case that was publicly told. Nobody understood what they were talking about. Our generation could not understand that because of sex you will die today. If the brother [Olikoye] who was minister of health could not convince his own brother [Fela] that HIV was real, then . . ." Femi laughed somewhat bitterly instead of finishing his sentence. "There were hardly any cases. The only case that was in the paper was my father. A lot of people were dying, but they were lying it was malaria or typhoid. Nobody told the truth. Nobody still tells the truth. It's still even a big taboo. Even worldwide, it's still a big taboo. It's not a subject that anybody really wants to talk about."

But the announcement that Fela's death resulted from HIV/AIDS cracked the silence in Nigeria and reverberated across the continent. Even if it did not immediately convince everybody that the disease was real or provide a deeper understanding of the epidemic, it allowed conversation to happen. People sat up. People started talking. A number of prominent activist organizations, such as Journalists Against AIDS, were founded at this moment to encourage more conversation about HIV/AIDS.

Death can advance quietly only so far before it inspires speech. The conversation develops slowly, beginning as an intense private reckoning that a person affected (not necessarily infected) by HIV has with himself or herself, before emerging in the public sphere.

For Samaila, the northern Nigerian HIV/AIDS activist and former policeman, the conversation started when his wife was hospitalized with end-stage AIDS. It was the same time he discovered that he too was HIV positive. "Saddiq, my oldest child, got to know when she was still in the hospital. Two weeks' stay is a very long time," he told me. "Saddiq's school was near the hospital, so he could come after school, still in his uniform. My daughter was too young. She couldn't comprehend. During that time, it was very hard for me and hard for them too, but it was then that I told him what was wrong with his mother. We were at home, in the house, sitting on the bed, when he asked me, 'Is my mother going to die?' I said, 'She may die.' Saddiq was around eleven or twelve when I found out I was HIV positive. He asked, 'Will you die too? Are you also going to die then, Daddy?' I had to tell him the truth. I said, 'I may die.'" He fell silent and crossed his arms over his chest. "Of course, at that time, I did not have the information I have now," he said, emerging from his recollections. "I thought God will take care of everything. If bad, it is the will of God. If good, it is also the will of God. I kept asking myself, 'What will happen to my children? What will become of them?' I grew to love them even more because I knew I would leave them. We would watch the television, walk around the countryside, sit on a stone and talk, explore their interests. But I kept asking myself, 'What will I do? How will I look for a cure?'"

He opened his palms to me and let them rest on his lap.

"I also decided to educate myself about HIV. I was reading a lot about HIV/AIDS. Anything I laid hands on about HIV/AIDS, I read. It was from the papers that I realized the federal government had planned to treat ten thousand people in the country. Also in the papers, I got to know about three people who were campaigning actively. Two of these people were also HIV positive like me, and their names always came out in the papers. After my retirement had been approved, I went to Lagos to claim my benefits. I took that opportunity to see those people. I went to see those people through an organization called Journalists Against AIDS. I followed an address that

I got from the newspaper, and I went to their office. They asked me to go back to where I was staying and start a support group for people living with AIDS, so that when the drugs come, it will be easy for them to get the required number.

"So I decided that certainly if I've got this information, I have to impart this information to other people. I started giving people information about HIV/AIDS, the stigma, drugs, positive living, and things like that within the communities in which I work—the Hausa Muslim communities of northern Nigeria. It was an uphill task getting to know other people who were HIV positive. People refused to come out. But by the end of the day, I was able to get ten, and then we started a support group. I went on television in my locality. I tried to organize workshops. Some of us took the bull by the horns and, as I said before, decided to come out public with our status and maybe in that way galvanize some sort of response from the government, philanthropists, and donors who could come to our aid. If we hid and the virus was not seen, if we didn't give a face to the virus, certainly there wouldn't be anything done on our behalf. And so some of us, including me, my humble self, decided to come out with our status."

After speaking with a number of people who have gone public with their HIV status, I realized that

Samaila's movement from internal contemplation to public disclosure is one that many people experience in their own ways. That moment of first disclosure brings an internal wrangling with the idea that HIV causes death and will cause one's own death, which after time can grow into a desire to understand whether this new force in life, HIV/AIDS, actually means life's end. This process usually occurs simultaneously with the heavy task of speaking of one's condition to family, friends, and loved ones, knowing that disclosure can have a profound emotional effect on the people who have been informed. Finally comes the realization that your story is a powerful tool if used publicly and communicated properly. But public communication is difficult for all who choose to engage in that conversation. It requires navigating the tension between the powerful negative messages about HIV/AIDS that already exist and the desire to spread new messages that humanize the epidemic.

Journalists Against AIDS has been a major force in shaping public discussion about HIV/AIDS in Nigeria. The group was founded shortly after Fela Kuti's death by the late Omololu Falobi, the former features editor at the popular Nigerian newspaper *Punch*. Its initial mission was to use journalism as a means for raising awareness about HIV/AIDS, but it has since grown into a major advocacy and capacity-building organization with programs that provide economic opportunities for people living with HIV/AIDS. At the group's headquarters in a house on a quiet side street in the Ogba area of Lagos, I met with a program officer named Jessam Nwaigbo, whose work focuses on evaluating media reporting on HIV/AIDS.

"For me, I pick up a newspaper and I see 'deadly scourge'—some say 'dreaded disease,' 'an AIDS victim languishing' or 'lamenting'—it gives me a very negative sense, and I might not want to read that further. Some say when writing about HIV, they use the scary red. We all know that the color red is danger. When it comes to HIV, you now use red and bold; so you're rather scaring me than passing off any useful information."

She took a moment to secure behind her ears her black and blond braids, which had come loose as she gestured passionately while she spoke. Every so often while emphasizing a point, she placed a palm on her heart, covering the silver design of her T-shirt.

"The people we are communicating with, they are a very large audience. You may not know who is picking up that magazine today. We are the third highest in terms of burden," she said, referring to the fact that Nigeria has the third largest population of HIV-positive people in the world. "A lot of people will be reading that newspaper. Your terms are not friendly. You would rather be reporting scary messages that will be scaring your audience rather than bring them forward to know their status. If they are reading issues that are so stigmatizing, they will say, 'Of what use I should know my status when I know that I am going to die,' or 'I don't have hope. There is nothing hopeful for me in this life.' We're not saying you should not say the truth, but people who have HIV—they are not victims. I hardly fall ill. I can stay throughout the year without falling ill. So how am I a victim? Do I run to you begging you for money or help? Did you rush me to the hospital or something? It's not a very friendly language. So we train the media on how to communicate this issue without using terminology that may be offensive."

Jessam's choice of work was the direct result of the negative conversation and messaging that she encountered when she first discovered her positive status in 2004. She heard people speaking about HIV/AIDS in her church, in the media. There was no question that the illness existed, but the level of judgment and stigmatization bothered her, as did the use of discussion about it as a tool to enforce existent moral norms. Her involvement with Journalists Against AIDS was a way of both renewing her commitment to life and reshaping the conversation that she heard happening around her.

"I wanted to do the work because I didn't want other people to pass through what I went through, both the psychological, the physical trauma, the emotional pain," she said as we sat in the darkened office conference room. The blinds were pulled shut over the window to block out the intense sun and keep the room cool. "I have been in that position where I thought probably dying should be the best option for me. And I overcame it, and I've met people in the course of my work who are saying, 'Ah, Jessie, do you think I can live? Do you think anything good can come of me? Don't you think I'm going to die tomorrow?' And I'm telling them, 'Is it a dead person who is talking to you? I am positive.' And they say, 'Are you sure, are you sure they did not give you money to stand in front of us? How can you be positive and you're looking good?' It's something that you ought to give back to society. Because I was given, I have to give back. I never can tell who is listening to me and will make a U-turn like I did. Real-life experiences goes a long way to combat the spread of HIV and mitigate the impact of AIDS."

"Real life" in the conversation about HIV/AIDS need not be limited to the experiences and stories of people living with the disease. It can also mean pulling the disease from the realm of idea, where it exists for most people, and molding it into language and a form to which people can relate. In Nigeria, broad-based social marketing done by NGOs like the Abuja-based Society for Family Health plays a large role in bringing the conversation about HIV/AIDS to the people through radio announcements in native tongues or pidgin English and posters that can be found in nearly every health center around the country. But even they would admit that such efforts are not nearly as effective in generating discussion and awareness as locally produced events and peer-to-peer interactions.

In May 2007, I flew from Abuja to Owerri in southeastern Nigeria to visit Felix, an HIV/AIDS program coordinator and activist I had met earlier that year at the national stakeholders conference in Abuja. He had already introduced me to Hope, one of the clients of his program, but this time my visit was to attend an AIDS Awareness Day program he had organized in his village just outside the city. He picked me up from the airport in a burgundy Toyota Corolla, its speakers blasting a man's falsetto voice crooning "You Give Me Fever."

When you meet Felix, you realize that everything about him is dramatic. His whole person seems carefully produced for maximum impact on whomever or whatever he meets. He has intense brown eyes that lock onto people and hold them captive. His deep voice, depending on his point, either rumbles into a heavy laugh or pinches into a brief squeak of concern. But it is his body language that is most convincing, his constantly moving hands in fists or palms as he speaks, his head cocked ever so quickly to the side, his brow furrowed when he makes a point that he wants you to find important. Felix had wanted to study acting in college, but his parents had pressured him to drop it. Acting is not generally considered a respectable profession in Nigeria, especially not for a first son and future family head. He ended up taking a degree in management technology. After graduating he worked a number of jobs, first producing documentaries for a rural branch of the national television authority, then working on a freight ship that hauled goods between West African port cities, and finally supervising the transportation of construction materials between cities in Nigeria. A run-in with armed robbers while on a job transporting rebar to Lagos led him to give up the trucker's life and focus on building a career in his hometown. That's how he came to work on youth programs and HIV/AIDS education.

He slowed after we passed through a four-way intersection with tall green grass growing at each of its corners. We slipped around a corner and pulled into an impromptu driveway created by tire tracks that had compacted the soft grass into the red mud and hardscrabble weeds. A large bungalow sat at the end of the path. Felix's father had started construction on the house but died before it was finished. Felix had scrimped and saved to complete it. His family didn't live there; they stayed in his apartment in town, but he kept the place because it gave him a presence in the village. I helped Felix drag an old diesel generator from a storeroom out onto the front porch. From there we carried it across the grass and loaded it into the car, which creaked and groaned under the weight.

Felix's village was like many others in the area. There was a paved street with low houses on either side, some behind concrete walls spiked with broken glass, the corrugated tin roofs just peeking over the wall's sparkling edge. Others were exposed, their front doors open and coughing out the young and old alike to sit in the hot sun, or swallowing them as they took respite from the heat. Off the paved street were dirt roads and paths people had trampled through the grass or bush. Villagers wearing colorful traditional fabrics walked home from church or from home to visit friends and relatives. All seemed unaware of the program Felix had created for them. In fact, the whole village appeared rather unconcerned with issues of HIV and AIDS until we rounded a bend in

the road and found a chaotic mass of teenagers milling about by the roadside seemingly without agenda,
some with laughter on their lips, others with more
serious faces, fully aware of this particular day's im-
portance. A group of older girls, dressed identically
in black skirts and tight white tops, tried desperately
to arrange young men and women into orderly lines
across the soft eroded red earth and in front of a low
bungalow that served as a village meeting place. The
building was much used but well cared for; it had
a fresh yellow coat of paint. Little children dangled
their feet from the low concrete walls of the veranda
as they watched the teenagers—their older siblings,
cousins, maybe even aunts and uncles—prepare for
the production.

When Felix finally pulled his car to a stop just
beyond the throng, a mighty shout rose up, as if a
great hero had arrived. Felix slipped into his role,
moving from group to group, offering greetings,
teasing and cracking jokes with kids, whose smiles
widened and eyes brightened in his presence. He was
electric, inspiring and controlling at the same time.
Within moments of his arrival, lines formed with the
loose regimentation of people unused to order. They
unfurled a white banner with red, blue, and green
lettering that encouraged the community to FIGHT
AIDS! A song erupted, led by a young woman; her

tight yellow shirt carried the slogan ZIP UP! It was a flirtatious appeal to abstinence.

"We are the world. We are its children," she sang. "We are the ones to make a better place, so let's fight AIDS now. We march in unity. Fighting H-I-V AIDS. We are the ones to make a brighter day, just you and me." The group behind her followed along in disorganized, democratic harmony.

From nowhere a young man appeared in the middle of the road, arm raised to his forehead in frozen salute. He wore a white cloth around his waist. The rest of his body was painted white from head to toe, and he wore black wraparound sunglasses. The word AIDS was painted in green across his chest, and when, after a long pause, he finally turned around, I saw that slogan found in so many social marketing campaigns—AIDS IS REAL—dripping down his back in the same green paint. He began a slow comical imitation of a soldier's march down a small stretch of road. The first regiment of youths followed him closely, holding candles in their hands with flickering flames that, in broad daylight, were almost invisible. The village road filled with young bodies, and the air grew heavy with a feverish call: "Fight fight fight AIDS!" The shrill voices of young women came to the point of cracking at the last minute, bolstered by young men's deep and rumbling call to arms: "Fight

fight fight AIDS!" Together they sang, "Today, today, tomorrow no more! If we fight AIDS today we
go fight am no more!" They clapped, stomped, and
ululated.

The whole group blobbed from one side of the
road to the other as curious drivers slowed to observe the commotion. I wasn't sure if the younger
marchers in the procession, the ten-year-olds, understood exactly why they were marching, but they
seemed overjoyed to be a part of something larger
than themselves. They weaved among older kids,
who seemed equally thrilled by the moment. Today
they could speak so freely about something so taboo.
As the group proceeded down the village road, the
noise they generated called people from their houses
to porches and front steps. A man appeared in his
doorway in green slacks and an undershirt, his eyes
dull with sleep. His two young daughters stood beside him in white dresses and head ties, all three
captivated by the shouting, singing youth. After a
moment, he smiled, clapped his hands, and shouted
words of encouragement. All along the road, this
scene repeated itself. Parents, grandparents, aunts,
uncles, cousins, friends: they appeared at windows
and on front lawns, on porches or in the cars sliding
by, and they cheered, they clapped, they honked. I
looked for Felix. He cautiously navigated the open

gutter's edge by the side of the road as he tried to provide subtle direction while letting the youths lead the way. His shirt clung to his body in places where the heat and humidity made him sweat.

"This is amazing!" I said to Felix when I managed to work my way through the mass of people over to him.

"My brother, eh!" was his only reply. He turned to face a car approaching the group and waved to the driver to slow down. "Have you seen this? Believe me. Young people are looking for something to say. They are looking for people to come out and lead them. They know that these problems are here, and they are looking for somebody that will come out and tell them, 'Let's start doing something to fight this problem.' This is creating a lot of awareness in the community. People who have seen are going to be touched by this. Young people who have been affected by HIV and AIDS are the people carrying out this message. Young people will learn from each other, and they will say, 'Who am I when my mates are actually on the road shouting anti-HIV/AIDS songs? Why wouldn't I join them?' And before you know it, behavior change starts to set in, gradually gradually."

Earlier, on the drive from the airport when he had first picked me up, Felix had said, "Young people tend to do things they hear from their mates. I'm a peer-education trainer for UNICEF, and when I go for peer-education training programs, I use myself as an example. I tell them they are very lucky, because all things I learned about sexuality, I learned on my own. My father never talked to me about it. My mother never talked to me about it. The real experience was when I visited a brothel. I had an inquisitive mind. I wanted to know exactly what it was like, because every day on my way to school, I would always pass through that brothel area, and you see young girls, you see guys drinking beer as early as seven thirty to eight in the morning. I was seeing people smoking, drinking—very rough faces—and I thought it was one wonderful thing. That first time I went, I felt like I was into something the big boys do. When I came out, I regretted the whole move. You know, sex is one thing; the excitement is that when you haven't done it, you haven't done it. There is vagina; you want to put your penis in it and know you're doing it. But by the time you know, you come, and you're like, 'Is this all? Is this all?' And you're paying money!

"I got gonorrhea and I didn't like it. When I was having pains, I didn't even go to my father. I didn't go to my mum. I went to my schoolmates. I went and talked to a young guy that was actually in my class. The guy was like, 'Don't worry! It's a very small thing!' He told me I should go and buy schnapps, kai-kai [a local moonshine], and drink a bottle of Coke filled up with kai-kai. I believed him. I took it, and it didn't stop. But where we were living, there was a pharmacist, and I went to him and said, 'Look. This is what is up.' The guy gave me an injection, and it stopped."

He smiled sheepishly and added, "So the concept of peer education actually comes from the fact that young people tend to influence each other more."

It's not a new concept. Popular culture, progressive attitudes, and new ideas around the world are usually generated by and promoted through the conversations and interactions of younger people. This often requires speaking loudly about precisely the things that make an older generation uncomfortable. Especially in Nigeria, youth voices often smash right into the stubborn will of the gerontocracy. Elders in our societies are treasured not only as people but also as textbooks of history, philosophy, ethics, and practical matters. Their life experience and their wisdom are the experience and wisdom of the whole community; therefore, they can readily, and in some cases justly, respond to agitating youth with the question "What do you know?" But a primary reason the HIV/AIDS epidemic exploded in Nigeria and the rest of sub-Saharan Africa is an unwillingness to seriously discuss issues that clearly affect youth. In many places around the world, the talk and action on HIV/AIDS and related issues, such as safe sex or treatment, have been driven by youth movements eager to bring attention to and find solutions for their concerns. The feedback, even if contentious or slow, often produces positive results.

When I asked Felix what the older people in the community would think about the day's events, he responded, "They are very happy about it. You're going to see them at the hall. They are all watching. They know that these problems are here, but they don't know how to tackle it. That's the problem. You see, when young people begin to do things themselves, the older people now come in. I have been able to sample their opinion, and I know that they are very much interested here. They like what is happening."

Indeed, when the youth march returned, the newly painted hall was filled with adults, who sat in the dimness fanning themselves. They were either unaware of or chose not to comment on the fact that the balloons dangling from the ceiling above them were actually inflated condoms. As each marcher entered the meeting hall, he or she dripped a bit of wax onto a concrete platform a single step off the ground, which served as a stage, then fixed his or her candle to the ground to the right of the platform until they had formed a large blazing AIDS ribbon. Then once reassembled onstage, they broke into religious praise songs. Even the elders clapped and lent their voices.

Suddenly a young man with a black Kangol cap turned backward and stepped toward the audience as the chorus behind him hushed down to a resonating hum. With an exaggerated strut, he approached a girl standing in the corner with close-cropped hair and prominent dimples on her nervous, smiling face. He peacocked around her, made sweet overtures, and stroked her cheeks, but she offered a forceful resistance. The audience chuckled knowingly as they gave the couple their full attention.

"I no want die. I no want catch AIDS!" the girl said loudly. "So make we wait until marriage or use condom."

The audience clapped while mm-hmm-ing and aha-ing at this message of responsibility appended to a plea for abstinence. Abstinence is, after all, the best way to prevent the spread of HIV and certainly an appreciated message in so religious a country as Nigeria. The skit also highlighted the complexities of messaging in communities that extol traditional values. In order to be effective, the conversation can push the limits only so far. As a messaging expert from the Society for Family Health explained to me, Nigerians are easily offended. As a country and within our separate cultural groups, we are still not ready to have explicit discussions about sex, as is done in the West. This is slowly changing, however, as new technologies allow a younger population access to a wider range of experiences and attitudes as well as more direct ways of communicating with one another.

In the darkness outside, thunder rumbled in the distance when the keynote speaker finally took the stage. He was a slight man with light brown skin, a pencil-thin mustache above his upper lip, and sweat soaking his clothes from the exertion of clapping and shouting in affirmation. His forehead was a glistening arc in the hall's dim light. For a moment before he spoke, the room was completely still. The chorus had stopped humming and stood silently behind him, next to the flickering candle AIDS ribbon. He wasn't from the village, and no one had seen him before. The way his white garment caught the candlelight, how his face shone, and the intensity of his gaze in that sliver of a moment before he opened his mouth made me feel that I had stumbled into a séance. In a sense, he was a seer because he was HIV positive, he said. The room hushed because none of us had known. You would never have been able to tell by looking at him.

"AIDS!" he shouted. "AIDS! Am I Doing Something? AIDS means ask yourself, 'Am I Doing Something?'"

Nigerians have a talent for inventing alternative meanings for acronyms. NEPA, the old Nigerian Electric Power Association, quickly became Never Expect Power Again and when renamed the Power Holding Corporation of Nigeria (PHCN) was popularly called Problem Has Changed Name. Despite the heat and the late hour, which had drawn the sound of tree frogs and crickets from the surrounding foliage, the audience perked up. "Am I doing something? Should I be doing something?" their newfound attention asked. "What can I do?"

The speaker stalked back and forth from one side of the stage to the other, fluidly switching between English and Igbo, tossing long strings of one language out to the audience along an accusatory finger and then punctuating them with short syllables from another, his "Yes oh!" and "Enh enh" mirrored in stereo sound by the villagers in front and the youthful chorus behind.

"AIDS. Am I Doing Something?" the speaker asked again.

"Am I Doing Something!" the audience responded for the last time before the speaker released them, putting an end to the night. The villagers filed away into the night, chattering about what they had just seen and experienced.

Felix and I hung around after the last of the villagers had departed. I helped him take down the balloons.

"I didn't actually know they were condoms," he said, laughing. "Can you imagine these youths?"

We finished by scraping the expended wax bits from the candlelight ribbon off the floor. Outside it was raining heavily. We stood at the door, watching the large drops batter the car windows and turn the red earth into a shifting mass.

I asked Felix what it means to "do something," and he said, "I often tell people, 'You know, you don't really need money to do the little things that you think are not really making some impact in people's lives.' But by the time you now do it a hundred times, two hundred times, and you put them together . . ." He trailed off. "All I know is that I'm actually doing this thing with my whole heart. I like what I'm doing. It's giving me joy. The little money that is going into my pocket, I am satisfied with. My salary is five thousand naira. There's a lot of my mates that are going home with one hundred thousand naira, working in better places. There's a lot of my mates that work for one business or another making their millions, but I think this is what my heart appreciates. I have a calling. Maybe I could say that this is a calling because I think my mind, my whole spirit, is appeased with what I'm doing. I feel I am impacting on somebody's life. I feel I am doing good. I'm in love with it."

"You're in love?" I was taken by his choice of words and the passion in his delivery, his insistence. His face was something different at that moment, his eyes wide, nostrils flared, his lips a thin, thoughtful line.

"Yes! You know when you are in love with a woman, you can actually do everything for that woman. You give the woman your time. You give the woman your life. You are patient. When you are in love with a woman, you will always want to do everything for the person. That is the way it is with me."

"Do you think programs like this actually change things?" I asked.

"I'm very hopeful," Felix said after some time. "I believe that the prevalence of it [HIV/AIDS] will still have to come down, but that will be dependent on the level we are taking this work to. We need to get more committed to this work. It has to go beyond rhetoric, just talking about it because you 'feel.' People have to be committed to it. People have to start realizing that local action, involving the community members, is what will really work. That's the only way it can be sustained. For people to really modify their behavior, you need to keep bombarding them with the same information, and as long as this information is coming from members of the same community, it makes a whole lot of sense."

The more we Nigerians—indeed, everyone in the world—speak about the disease, the more it weaves its way into everyday life. It begins to exist not just as a topic of discussion planted by public health officials and activists, but also as a genuine driver of and topic in our cultural expression. It appears in the films we watch, in the art we produce, and in the music we make.

For Femi Kuti, that HIV/AIDS should find its way into his music and artistic expression was part of a natural evolution. I first saw him perform live at a Boston nightclub in 2001, on my nineteenth birthday. Watching him perform with his Positive Force band and dancers is an amazing experience. His set that night was intense, fast paced, with frenetic drums beating the polyrhythms characteristic of Afro-beat and aggressive horns complementing his saxophone and singing. It was impossible to remain still. His music filled you up and made your body twitch and gyrate. It made you sweat—especially his song "Stop AIDS"—and only afterward did you realize what you had just been listening to.

With music designed to move your body in a way that suggests sex and lyrics designed to move your mind by expressing the fear, confusion, and hope associated with that activity in a world with HIV/AIDS, the song seeps into your consciousness in a way that direct messaging never could.

When I spoke with Femi about the song almost ten years later at his Shrine, he said, "Every night, even to now, I always make sure I play that number. The thing about music is you know that sometimes you don't have to say anything. You just give it a title. Just give it a title like 'Stop AIDS.' Even if I didn't sing any lyrics, just because of the music, everybody would know that it's about AIDS. It becomes a slang."

"So do you consider yourself an activist?" I asked him.

"Why are you calling me an activist?" he said. "It doesn't make sense. If you are concerned about mankind, they say you are a humanitarian. These are just stupid titles people give themselves because they want to be important. 'Oh, I'm a humanitarian. Oh, I'm an activist.' If you pick up a gun, you become a rebel or a terrorist. We just like titles. I just did or do what I felt I should do. I don't think I'm an activist. I'm just human."

HIV/AIDS is part of the human experience, part of our cultural experience. AIDS is everywhere. The last time I flew out of the Lagos airport, a friend and I noticed a poster hanging on a wall near the security checkpoint. In bright red letters, it read AIDS! NOW THAT WE HAVE YOUR ATTENTION, HAVE A SAFE FLIGHT AND REMEMBER, PLAY SAFE. It was an interesting display—all the more so because of its total irreverence. The conversation is developing slowly and organically—sometimes in the wrong direction—but always in the direction of more noise. The more noise we make about it, the more real HIV/AIDS becomes. The more real AIDS becomes, the more we consider it an aspect of our existence that we can engage with rather than an evil to run away from. That is the first step in treating the epidemic.

HEALING

The first time I visited Doc's clinic, I was amazed by how little there was inside. The one-story building featured nearly empty room after nearly empty room. In the lobby, our footsteps echoed against walls covered by a few instructional posters—how to breast-feed, how to do oral rehydration therapy—but there wasn't much else besides a few empty wooden benches that lined the walls. The exam rooms had old tables with rusted legs and foam padding pushing through cracks in their vinyl upholstery. There was a birthing room populated only by a bed frame, no mattress on its sagging springs. A storeroom with a few bottles on otherwise barren shelves served as a pharmacy. Doc said very little as we moved from room to room, pointing only to the items that would identify the purpose of each space—a broken operating table, nonfunctioning surgical lamps, a portable autoclave for sterilizing the few instruments he had at his disposal. When we finished the tour, the cavernous lobby was still empty. The room was quiet. Doc sighed with relief. There were no patients. It was only then that I realized that a number of the clinic's windows were missing windowpanes.

"This is where you work," I said to Doc.

He laughed the way he usually does when he considers something beyond explanation, and then he ushered me out to the front steps. "It's cooler out there," he said.

We sat on the building's steps just in front of the ramp that gave ambulances easy access to the triage rooms and lobby. Without patients that day, there wasn't very much to do but sit and wait for a government official Doc had invited to tour the clinic in hopes of convincing him to provide funds for its upkeep, possibly even an upgrade. He wasn't holding his breath. He had invited the man a number of times before, waited for hours, and not seen anyone. In fact, Doc had been waiting for four years, and still some of the windows lacked glass panes, the pharmacy was understocked, and the exam rooms were short on supplies. This, he told me, was the nature of health care in a resource-poor setting: you provide whatever care you can with the tools at your disposal. Sometimes he used money from his own salary, roughly four hundred dollars a month, to buy the necessary items for patient care, but that was when the state government remembered to pay him. It was immensely frustrating, he said. When he'd first arrived, he often thought of leaving, but now his random posting here as a young doctor just after he finished his internship had become a mission to bring adequate health care to the thousands of people living in the area. A large part of his work involved tackling the HIV/AIDS epidemic in the community.

"I started campaigning right through the time I came to serve," he said as we sipped from the now warm bottles of water I had carried with me from his house just down the road from the clinic. "I used HIV/AIDS awareness as my community development project," he said, explaining that a project was a requirement for everyone doing the mandated year of national service. He had started by organizing meetings in village squares, where he would educate men and women about its presence in the community and the methods of transmission and prevention, and since then he had added formal workshops for the villagers on HIV/AIDS, as well as a community health worker program to make home visits to people too weak or too remote to access the clinic.

"I didn't even know the significance of what I was doing. I didn't know the HIV incidence was high. I was just doing it out of somebody who had the energy to do something," he said. "Then I started seeing cases in the hospital. I remember there was a guy that came. He was almost my age. He tested positive, and it was very difficult to tell him because I don't have the drugs to help them. I don't have antiretroviral therapy. Assuming there is treatment available, I would say, 'Ah, don't worry about it!' And when I'm saying it, I would say it with full authority. 'You see this treatment? Once you take it, it's going to help you.' But sometimes when there is no help, you can only give supportive therapy and encourage elements of healthy, positive living—nutrition, take care of themselves more, any time they feel any symptoms, they should come to the hospital for treatment of opportunistic infections. If it's possible, I can also refer them to the government treatment program that is in the city. But most of them cannot afford the transportation cost."

He scuffed at a mud stain on the concrete steps with his sandal and rubbed his thighs with his hands.

"It was actually after that time I intensified. I moved even beyond education. I started doing trade-justice advocacy for access to treatment, because I knew it was crucial if people are going to get the message. It has transformative effects when people see hope, when they know that even if we are infected, we can still live. When people are down with AIDS, if you want to help them, you give them antiretrovirals. That's the only thing that can change their lives."

He rummaged through a folder of papers he carried with him, presumably documents for the visiting official. He produced a pamphlet from Paul Farmer's Boston-based international health organization, Partners in Health. On the cover were two juxtaposed photographs, one of an emaciated person with body sores, pustules, and a vacant stare, the other of a muscular man with a firm stance, wide smile, and bright eyes. "Can you believe it's the same patient, same person?" he said, pointing. "This is the magic of antiretroviral drugs."

HIV/AIDS is a treatable disease. It does not yet have a cure. It still causes many deaths in sub-Saharan Africa each year. But this does not mean the HIV virus is invincible. The HIV/AIDS epidemic in Africa can be brought under control. For the first time in the history of the African epidemic, the number of new infections most recently recorded has dropped by 20 percent since 1999. The annual number of AIDS-related deaths in sub–Saharan Africa has also decreased by about 20 percent since 2004. In Nigeria, although there has not yet been a decrease in the number of new HIV/AIDS infections or deaths, the numbers are not rising. This progress, however incremental, is the result of the complicated process of balancing large-scale health initiatives that target the general public with small-scale individualized treatment for people living with HIV/AIDS. One of the main tools in reducing the scope of the epidemic is the antiretroviral medication that Doc mentioned. These drugs can have dramatic effects on the health and quality of life of individuals living with HIV/AIDS, and in so doing, can also reduce the broader impact of the epidemic.

Antiretrovirals, commonly known as ARVs (or antiretroviral therapy [ART]), are a class of drugs that can stop the entry of the HIV virus into cells, the successful production of its genetic material once inside cells, and the assembly of the proteins that make up the HIV virus structure. ARVs keep the HIV virus at bay in a person's body, allowing his or her immune system time to recover and prevent the myriad infections that constitute AIDS. The drugs also reduce the amount of virus in a person's blood and body fluids, making him or her much less likely to pass the virus on to others. The first ARV, zidovudine, also known as azidothymidine (AZT), was developed in the United States in 1987. Its introduction completely changed the way the Western world dealt with HIV/AIDS as a disease and an epidemic. The initial treatments with early ARVs like AZT required patients to take large numbers of pills on a complicated schedule, often causing a number of unpleasant side effects, such as persistent nausea, diarrhea, and changes in metabolism and physical appearance. But no longer was HIV/AIDS considered a death sentence; no longer would it plow through a population unchecked.

By the time the extent of the African HIV/AIDS epidemic became clear, new drugs had been developed. Combination therapy with different types of ARVs reduced the number of pills needed and increased the effectiveness of the treatment. Now an HIV-positive person on ARVs can expect to live for years, possibly even long enough to die from something unrelated to HIV/AIDS. These drugs are powerful and effective, but they are not cheap. In the United States, without subsidies, the average yearly cost for a person taking ARVs can top ten thousand dollars. Luckily, in the United States and other nations with mature health systems, the cost of treatment can be subsidized. In sub-Saharan Africa, where the epidemic is at its worst and many of the HIV positive live on less than two dollars a day, people can ill afford the cost of treatment, and governments saddled with many other pressing issues cannot fully subsidize treatment. For this reason, until very recently, treatment with ARVs was not an option for most Africans living with HIV/AIDS.

The fact that the inability to afford treatment has

had such a profoundly exacerbating impact on the African HIV/AIDS epidemic has led some to suggest that the epidemic's root cause is not just a tiny virus, but also the larger systemic problem of extreme poverty. Individuals who cannot afford ARVs often see their HIV infection progress to full-blown AIDS. Poor countries with underfunded health systems are usually unable to provide the proper care and treatment to their citizens that would prevent that progression. The continent of Africa, which unfortunately is home to a large number of the world's poorest countries, experiences a double hit: poverty worsens the HIV/AIDS epidemic, and the epidemic worsens poverty.

"You know, it's so unfortunate the way things are, that Africa has been caught up with this AIDS stuff, and it further paints the continent in a bad light," Doc said. "It's not as if Africans do things that every other person is not doing, but just because of some other factors: there is already poverty; a lot of people are not educated [about the virus]. Those things make the virus spread fast. I think it's just unfortunate for us. And because we were already poor, the virus made us poorer, and made it more difficult to respond to the whole thing."

For many activists like Doc, the link between HIV/AIDS and poverty provides both cause for anger and an avenue for action, particularly concerning access to treatment. It starts with a question that Doc asked as we waited for the government official to arrive: "It's just in 2001 that people started talking about treatment in Africa. How is it possible that years after people were getting treatment in developed countries, they still thought it was not feasible for countries in Africa to have access to treatment?"

For Doc and many other HIV/AIDS activists, the answer was that Westerners had failed to see people in Africa with HIV/AIDS as similar to ourselves and thus deserving of proper medical care. For Africans who have HIV/AIDS, the marginalization is twofold. First comes the stigma. Next is the general marginalization of the continent resulting from poverty. It is by now a truism that the global poor are castaways without access to the same resources enjoyed by those with means. Their needs are neglected, their fundamental human rights often ignored. Being African and HIV positive elicits intentional and unintentional neglect in the domestic and international spheres. The option of mass treatment was not seriously pursued, and emphasis was placed on programs to prevent those without HIV/AIDS from contracting the virus. For some activists, the greater emphasis on prevention was tantamount to writing off as lost the very large population of marginalized people who were already positive. They turned an intellectual debate among public health professionals about where to best invest limited resources— prevention versus treatment—into an urgent human rights issue. Not providing treatment to those most vulnerable and least able to afford it was portrayed as a statement by African and international leaders that HIV-positive Africans did not have a fundamental right to health. By recasting the lack of treatment in human rights terms, activists transformed the HIV/ AIDS epidemic into more than just a health issue; it became a political issue with increasingly political and economic solutions.

From Cape Town to Abuja, indeed throughout the whole continent, organizations like the Treatment Action Campaign of South Africa or Doc's very own Physicians for Social Justice have tied together access to treatment, political activism, economics, and human rights. They continue to stress these links today. By putting political pressure on governments and social pressure on the makers of HIV/ AIDS medications, they developed a plan of action to stem the epidemic with language that emphasized the right to proper care through the provision of ARV treatment, the strengthening of health systems, and the creation of domestic and international bodies with the power to tackle the issue. The 2001 Abuja

Declaration on HIV/AIDS, Tuberculosis, and Other Related Infectious Diseases, signed by African heads of state at a summit in Nigeria's capital, is a direct result of this push to make treatment available to all. In addition to formally recognizing the severity of the HIV/AIDS epidemic, the declaration also called for increased domestic health care budgets with funds specifically allocated for HIV/AIDS prevention and treatment and the "creation of a Global AIDS Fund capitalized by the donor community to the tune of US $5–10 billion accessible to all affected countries to enhance operationalization of Action Plans, including accessing Anti-retroviral programmes in favour of the populations of Africa." At the international level, this resulted in the creation of the Global Fund to Fight AIDS, Tuberculosis, and Malaria; increased focus on HIV/AIDS from economically oriented donor organizations, like the World Bank; and most recently and perhaps most effective in providing ARV therapy to many people throughout the continent, the creation of the U.S. President's Emergency Plan for AIDS Relief, commonly known as PEPFAR.

At the domestic level in Nigeria, the Abuja declaration bolstered recently created governmental structures to handle the HIV/AIDS emergency. The National Agency for the Control of AIDS (NACA), established in February 2000 and headquartered in

Abuja, was to handle Nigeria's federal government response to the epidemic, while the states formed SACAs—state agencies for the control of AIDS—to coordinate the various local responses. While imperfect, the result has been an improved focus on the epidemic in Nigeria with better strategies for prevention and greatly improved access to treatment for people living with HIV/AIDS. The change is incremental, but each year the cooperation of international and domestic partners brings services to an increasing number of people.

In June 2007, I visited the Lagos State Agency for the Control of AIDS (LSACA), headquartered at the Lagos General Hospital. The hospital sits right in the center of Lagos Island, steps away from the water, separated from the marina by a traffic-choked highway. It is a tightly packed collection of old, worn buildings squeezed between a number of iconic skyscrapers housing some of Nigeria's largest banks and industries. The LSACA office was an even smaller building, possibly an old block of servants' quarters, that suffered between two large wings of the hospital, right next to a deafening standby generator. I met an official there who agreed to speak with me, anonymously on account of his sensitive government position.

He was in his early forties and had hints of gray,

even on his closely shaved head. He spoke slowly and with the slight British accent belonging to a certain class of Nigerians. In what he called a previous life, six years earlier, he had been an obstetrician at a government hospital.

"I had this image of being able to save people's lives and bring babies into the world, make everyone happy, deal with complicated cases. And I was doing a bit of that, but a lot of the women were coming when it was too late to help them, and you ended up bringing out almost as many dead babies as you did live ones," he said as he leaned back in a black swivel office chair and crossed his legs. We sat in a conference room with a noisy air conditioner circulating the musty smell of old files stacked upon files against the walls. The table in front of us took up most of the space, making it hard to move around the room without bumping knees or feet against the furniture. "I wanted to do good, but I also wanted to feel good, and somehow it didn't all come together. At one point, I was just going to quit and get into a private setting or go into something entirely different from medicine." He chuckled softly and spread his arms toward the chaos. "I ended up here. And the first few days it was just paper around me, and I thought, *What the hell did I let myself in for?* Files, papers, I don't know squat about that kind of stuff.

"I think we're making quite a lot of difference," he said. "When this first agency started, the response to HIV and AIDS had just started, so everything was new. I think we've managed to organize things in quite a decent way. We're not where we want to be—I know that. We're slowly going, but on a good path, I think."

It had been an intense and not altogether pleasant beginning. Many people considered the agency yet another level of bureaucracy destined to siphon precious money meant for Nigerian citizens in need. They also wondered why it wasn't doing more, and doing it faster. The agency lacked adequate funding to properly execute both prevention and treatment programs, but more recently it had gained the confidence of the general public and people living with HIV/AIDS because of increased funding from international donor agencies. The staff had put the money to work by expanding counseling and testing programs and improving access to treatment.

"Because treatment is available free, counseling and testing is available free, many people believe in us more," he said. "The bulk of my work, my goal really, is to see that the people who are not positive remain not positive, the people who are positive and need treatment get access to treatment, and for the people who don't need treatment, to delay the time at which they would need treatment, and then to mitigate the impact on the lives of those who are positive and their families. But not to mitigate it in a way that problems they had even before they are positive then get solved. Hell, I have problems, and they are not going to go away tomorrow. There is nothing that says a positive person's problems should go away tomorrow."

"What do you mean?" I asked. I was somewhat taken aback. His frankness was very uncharacteristic for a government official.

"I'm the kind of person who likes to say things as I see them. I think that positive people need to get off their butts and stop thinking that everything has to fall into place for them just because they're positive. They need to take more responsibility for their lives. Responsibility equals asking to be treated like an equal. I don't know if I'm getting the picture across. I can't say to you, 'I'm blind. I don't want you to treat me different from you,' but say, 'Oh. Any time I want to cross the road, walk me across.' And when we sit down about something, I say, 'Why are you treating me as if I have a disability or [as] if I'm different from you?' No. If I want to be independent, I should cross the road by myself. There are a lot of people that are not positive in this country that cannot eat three square meals. There are a lot of people that are not positive in this country that are ill and need to pay for their treatment because there is no proper health insurance scheme. There are a lot of people that are not positive and need to work very hard to achieve what they achieve."

In the six years he had been at LSACA, he had encountered a number of HIV-positive people who had tried to take advantage of the increased funding for HIV/AIDS-related work. Others, he said, had developed a sense of entitlement that he saw as undermining the institutions set up to protect their interests and ensure equal standing in the eyes of the general public.

"They come at you with an attitude sometimes like, 'Hey, I'm positive. You guys are here because of me.' People want you to give them things just because they are positive; they want you to do things for them just because they are positive. They want everything to be free just because they are positive. It doesn't work like that." He sat up and stopped his chair from its squeaky rocking. "We are trying to tell people, 'Don't discriminate, don't stigmatize positive people, because they are no different from you.' Let's say that positive people are like you and me, no different; let that be across the board. I'm here to see that they get access to treatment, they are not stigmatized, they are treated like human beings. I'm not really here to make sure their rent is paid, because people who don't have HIV are having problems paying their rent. 'I'm positive—so what?' That's the message we're all trying to spread: 'People are people, whether or not they have HIV.'"

His blunt words reflect both frustration and a deep practical commitment to restoring the fundamental equality of people living with HIV/AIDS. It avoids pity and the patronizing attitudes that sometimes affect those more distant from the realities on the ground. If people are people, then efforts against the disease and its epidemic should seek to restore their functionality as people. This is the role of medication. It allows the body to operate. It eases the burden of illness. It removes the physical signs of disease. It abates the fear of imminent death. Treatment saves lives, but a solution to this epidemic requires more.

I didn't know it at the time, but around the corner from the LSACA office was a large ARV treatment facility. Four years later, I found myself in front of the building, ready for a whole day of interviews with people receiving treatment. It is not an easy place to find; rather, it's the sort of place you would need to know is there before you could locate it. Yet it is a stop for thousands of people who are receiving drugs that will prevent their HIV from turning into full-blown AIDS. The facility was in what appeared to be a large storage space with exposed steel beams and visible wooden frames supporting a corrugated tin roof. The open floor had been sectioned into consulting rooms by flimsy plywood dividers. Privacy was minimal. Patients sat on uncomfortable wooden benches, apparently bored stiff. They fanned themselves with bits of paper and open palms while waiting, and waiting, and waiting, to see a doctor, nurse, or counselor to discuss their lab results and treatment regimens.

It was here that I met Angie, a twenty-eight-year-old woman with a waiflike figure. She wore skinny jeans with heels, and her lipstick had the faintest hint of glitter. She bounced her legs nervously as we sat in metal chairs squeezed into an exam room now used for storage. It was crowded with extra file cabinets and dust-covered standing fans.

In 2005 Angie had just finished college and started work when her life changed. She tested positive for HIV. "I was supposed to get married, but I've missed that," she said. "You know what it is like when you see your wedding gown, you share clothes to people, and the guy just walks out?" She let out a bitter laugh and shook her head. Her earrings made a tinkling sound as tiny metal rods knocked against each other. "I was actually working in a bank, and you know, it's very difficult at times to say you want to go out of the office. At the office, I couldn't really tell them I had HIV. I told them I had TB and I had to be away from work for treatment. They actually wanted to treat me in the office, but I didn't allow them. In the office, they now found out or something, because they stopped paying me for that eight months while I was receiving my treatment." She sighed heavily as her eyes filled with tears. She wiped the corners of her eyes with her fingertips and tried to breathe deeply to calm herself. "I'm sorry," she said.

I put a hand on her knee and said, "Angie, it's OK."

When she brought her hands away from her face, her fingertips were stained with mascara.

"I've been taking these drugs for . . . how many years?" she said. "And I thought I'd outgrown it, but the anger is just starting again. Right now I don't know how to continue. When I was working, I didn't really have much problems with my health. It was easy for me to manage myself. I work. I eat well. I do anything I want to do. I didn't have any complaints. But right now I have different complaints, so I now know one of the problems that makes people to die from this: you think. Thinking is the major problem—when I think of so many things I've lost. Because I started thinking, my CD4 count has dropped. I just have to stop. I was feeling like a strong woman before, but now I don't know. I feel very very depressed. I feel very, very trapped. I'm in a cage right now. I'm just living life as it comes. I'm just there. I'm very lonely."

Angie was a physically healthy HIV-positive young woman, taking her medications consistently and showing up for all of her follow-up care, but something was not right. She was not completely herself, not fully restored. With such great focus placed on procuring drugs and strengthening or building the health systems to deliver treatment to large numbers of people affected by the epidemic, it can be easy to forget that treatment alone does not make a person better. Nor will treatment by itself change the course of the epidemic. To really make an impact, we need to move beyond a focus on providing treatment and toward the idea of healing.

At the induction ceremony for my medical school class, where we incoming future doctors were given our brand-new white coats by the dean of students, the keynote speaker, writer and physician Abraham Verghese, made the point that anyone can be taught the principles of treating illness, the technical aspects of care—what medicine to prescribe and how much, the surgical techniques necessary to remove a tumor or repair an aneurysm—and that these skills are extremely important, indeed central, to the practice of medicine. But healing, he suggested, is something different. Healing is that ineffable something that happens between the person providing care and the patient, which may improve life, even in the absence of a treatment that leads to a cure. Healing requires more than technical proficiency; it requires an ability to connect to another person. Healing requires compassion, "a shared sense of humanity," and the ability to see another's pain as "the kind of thing that could happen to anyone, including oneself insofar as one is a human being."

In other words, we have our drugs and our prevention campaigns, but that is not enough. To restore basic functionality, we must focus on providing treatment to people living with HIV/AIDS, just as it is necessary that we develop tools to treat the broader epidemic. But we also need to focus on restoring the human connection that the disease tears asunder. As a nurse and HIV counselor I spoke with told me, "When you have HIV, you're the type of person that is supposed to be loved by people. There is need they have that love, because when there is not love, the tension will be too much and they can easily die— not from the sickness but the heartsickness."

It is no surprise, then, that many people with HIV/AIDS find comfort not only in the fact that medication will help them live longer, but also in the connections made through support groups and associations, and through work that reconnects them to their communities. As Samaila Garba, the activist and former police officer, put it, "I would have been a different story without the ARVs. I would have been talked of as 'he was,' not 'he is.' I was about to die just like that. I saw death coming, and then I saw it pass me by, so to speak. If you entered an airplane, and the airplane crashed and every other person died but you didn't die—you came out and escaped—you are going to have an entirely different perspective on life. And that is the perspective that I have now. There are finer, more beautiful things in life that we have looked at but we have not been able to see, simply because we didn't place any value on life. It is not the amassing of wealth, the mad rush for material things, the mad rush for academic laurels and other things. That will pass by. I have seen amassing wealth or things that other people attach to life as important as nonsense and useless. I now have time to understand people. I now have time to think twice before dealing with people. My relationship with my community, with my neigh-bors, even my children, has been greatly affected by the fact that I was about to die and didn't die. I have realized that the greater things of life are love, being useful, being counted, and making a positive impact on other people's lives."

It should not be a one-way street. The onus of promoting this shared sense of humanity should not rest solely on those who are HIV positive. Those of us who are not HIV positive must understand that people with HIV/AIDS are people, and this should be reflected in our actions and relationships.

I know a barber named Gabriel, who told me about a friend of his who contracted HIV. While others ran away from the man on account of his illness, Gabriel stayed with him and took care of him until he died. When I asked him why, he said, "I have that spirit of love that sees every human being as part of me, that spirit of love that you see your fellow man as part of you."

He spoke as we sat outside his barbershop in Abuja late at night, at a table placed just by the roadside. He had stretched his long legs out between us, crossed them and slumped into the fatigue of a day's worth of standing on his feet cutting hair. He played with his sweatpants as we spoke, zipping and unzipping the side pockets or twirling the waist tie.

"At that time, HIV wasn't that popular like now. Those years, it's something that just started, and people knew that this thing kills and there's no cure—automatically no cure. People were not open to such information about HIV, and that was the first reason for discrimination. When somebody has it, you will find your way, you will not even come to him again because you heard he has HIV. You will just discriminate the person, meaning that you will not relate with the person."

"But you stayed with your friend," I said.

"I did that because I found out that you cannot continue to say that you put a condition to love somebody. I can love anybody. I love everybody. They may call you prostitute. They may call you armed robber. Whatever it is! Love you! Love you! I'm being serious. I'm being sincere. Believe me. If you don't have this character, meaning that you see beyond certain things, you will not be free to live as free man. But when you have this mentality, this spirit at work in you, there is nowhere you cannot stay because you will always have people around you, and those people are your brother and sisters. You don't see them as stranger or foreigner. You can't meet good people by limiting yourself. You can't go further in life when you have those limitations," he said. "I don't have that idea of separation or discrimination. It's not a part of me."

In the quivering fluorescent light, a squadron of insects flickered against its harsh illumination. The night air, warped by the heat, encouraged slowness, silence. He looked at me, his eyes wide and glowing, and said, "I am ready to cross any boundary."

If this virus and its epidemic are to be contained, the strategy must be one that in word and deed re-affirms human connections on individual and international levels. We must endeavor to cross the boundaries we have set up that separate HIV-positive people from HIV-negative people. Then will the healing begin.

AIDS IS NOT MY IDENTITY

The global HIV/AIDS epidemic is now more than thirty years old, and in the absence of a miracle cure, it will grow older. In its short time with us, HIV/AIDS has become a powerful force, and not just because it has caused millions of deaths. It is more than just a biological occurrence. It is a major cultural event of the modern era that has reshaped the relationships that individuals, countries, and even whole continents have with one another. It has come to represent the continent of Africa and the people living in it, limiting their abilities to define their own identities as individuals interacting with a challenging and complex world.

One of the last people I spoke with in Nigeria was a family friend, Paul Nwabuikwu, a former editorial board member of the Nigerian newspaper the *Guardian*. His editorials and opinions are highly regarded by many Nigerians, and he has written extensively on a number of social and political topics, including HIV/AIDS. "I'm very uncomfortable with the way AIDS has morphed from being something that started in the West to being another face

of Africa. Just like hunger. Just like political insta-
bility. Just like poverty," he said. "I'm very uncomfortable with that transformation. As a Nigerian, as
an African, I have to make the point that, yes, I
understand this is real, but it's not my identity. I re-
fuse to accept it. It's a disease that affects everybody,
but it's not my identity." Because Paul does not have
HIV, one might be tempted to dismiss his statement
as the thoughts of someone who doesn't really know
what it's like to live with the disease, but his words
reflect an attitude apparent in all the people I met,
HIV positive or not, while researching and writing
this book: HIV is not the entirety of who I am as
a person; it is not the entirety of who we are as a
country or continent.

The people who shared their stories with me
have approached HIV/AIDS and its impact in different ways. Some, like Hope, have sought a quiet
existence full of routine, family, and daily concerns,
of which HIV/AIDS is one of many. Others, like
Samaila Garba or Jessam Nwaigbo, have been more
vocal in a quest to combat the stigma that limits the
opportunities of HIV-positive people in Nigeria and
the rest of the world. Many have tried to provide care
and emotional support to people living with HIV/
AIDS. The driving force for everyone, it seems, is a
profound sense of commitment to the idea of a com-

mon humanity. Their lives, their stories, and their actions are an acknowledgment that, disease or no disease, we are all fundamentally the same. We are all human.

HIV/AIDS, however real, cannot change that.

ACKNOWLEDGMENTS

Our *Kind of People* has been a long time in the making. There are many who have helped me along the way.

First and foremost, I owe much to all of you who, over the past few years, were kind and trusting enough to share some intensely personal stories with me. Many of you will remain anonymous, but your words, your thoughts, your experiences are this book. Thank you.

To Dr. Chukwumuanya Igboekwu: over the past few years, since we first spoke about HIV/AIDS in Nigeria, you have become a close friend. I am very grateful to you for your thoughts and your guidance on how to make this book a reality.

To Samaila Garba: I am full of admiration for the work that you have done. Your warmth and enthusiasm have always been an inspiration. I hope that in some small way this book embodies the spirit with which you approach your work.

I would be remiss if I did not thank the following people for the help and insight they have provided: Rolake Odetoyinbo, Helen Epstein, Paul Nwabuikwu, Femi Kuti, Jessam Nwaigbo-Okoi Edet, Ibrahim Umoru, Femi Adegoke (and everyone he introduced me to), Frank, and my friends at NACA and the Ministry of Health.

To my agents, Jeff and Tracy (and Andrew), and my editors, Tim and Eleanor, thank you for your encouragement and your willingness to stick with this project despite my taking a "little" detour through medical school. I'd say I owe you one, but I actually still owe you one, so we'll just skip that.

To my research assistants: Desta, Katharine, and Rachael. Thank you for all your help with the nitty-gritty.

To my friends who have provided both moral and material support: I would not be where I am without you.

Emma: not only did you read this draft in its original form, you also housed me for the summer it took to turn it into something readable. I am so grateful for your help and friendship. Thank you, Tim and Eliot, for your kindness as well.

ACKNOWLEDGMENTS

Larissa: thank you for all the lunches where you listened to me drone on about this book and my anxieties. Thank you for a thorough reading of my first draft and your equally thorough commentary. Thanks to you and Philip for housing me this summer. Last but not least, thanks to the girls for taking care of Maximus while I was away.

Ian: WLA. This book has words—real words—because of you. Thank you for all the time you spent wrestling with not so very good drafts as though they were your own work.

Thenji: your cover, your thoughts on my chapters, and your appreciation of what it means to try to tell the right stories about our continent are all such a big part of what this book is. Thank you.

Elliot: you are one of the few people who really understand what writing means to me and what I hope to do with it. Thank you for listening and for reading.

Meehan: working with you was such a pleasure that I looked forward to our many therapy—I mean editing—sessions at your house as the highlight of my week. You have a mind for structure like I have never known and such a wonderful way of being brutally honest with the utmost love. I would not have made it through this book without you.

The Robins: consider this as me thanking each

of you separately but wanting so badly to be able to call you "the Robins." In completely different ways you have been a source of perspective, wisdom, and support.

Megan: your research was always on point, your transcriptions incredible, and your stories—priceless.

Ragamuffin, Louisa, Jennifer S., Steph, Julie, Rebekah, Jennifer B., Manka, Mary: thank you for your support, advice, and eyes.

Nina: you were there at the beginning, when this book was just an idea I pestered you with—constantly. Thank you for the poster, and thank you for still being there.

To my family: Uncle Chi-Chi and Auntie Uju (Lagos just isn't the same without you) and of course to Daddy, Mommy, Onyi, Andrew, Oke, Uch, Milo, and now Adaora. I love you all.

NOTES

AIDS IS REAL

25   American Invention to Discourage Sex: Ogoh Alubo, "Breaking the Wall of Silence: AIDS Policy and Politics in Nigeria," *International Journal of Health Services* 32 (2002), no. 3: 551–66.

26   "wipe out entire generations": "Nigeria: Statement by His Excellency President Olusegun Obasanjo," 57th United Nations General Assembly, United Nations Secretariat, New York, Sept. 15, 2002, www.un.org/webcast/ga/57/statements/020915nigeriaE.htm.

27   4 percent of Nigeria's population: *National HIV/AIDS & Reproductive Health Survey*, Federal Ministry of Health, Abuja, 2006.

27   34 million positive people: *AIDS Epidemic Update 09* (Geneva: Joint United Nations Programme on HIV/AIDS, Nov. 2009), http://data.unaids.org/pub/report/2009/jc1700_epi_update_2009_en.pdf; *UNAIDS World AIDS Day Report 2011* (Geneva: Joint United Nations Programme on HIV/AIDS, 2011), www.unaids.org/en/media/unaids/contentassets/documents/unaidspublication/2011/JC2216_WorldAIDSday_report_2011_en.pdf; *National Policy on HIV/AIDS*, Federal Government of Nigeria, 2009, http://nigeria.unfpa.org/pdf/ntpol.pdf.

34   "worst years of my life": Fred Adegbulugbe, "I Waited Four
       Years for Death," interview of Rolake Odetoyinbo, *Punch*
       (Nigeria), Feb. 8, 2009, http://archive.punchontheweb
       .com/Articl.aspx?theartic=Art20090208193851.

35   "I didn't know much about HIV": Jemi Ekunkunbor, "HIV
       Made Me Feel Ugly and Battered but No More—Rolake
       Odetoyinbo Nwagwu," interview, *Vanguard* (Nigeria), Aug.
       1, 2004, www.impactaids.org.uk/newsletter/Newletter_Ar
       chive/VAN–1.htm.

35   "wasn't in a hurry to kill me": Adegbulugbe, "I Waited."

37   "I don't want to go out and look like HIV": Ekunkunbor,
       "HIV Made Me Feel Ugly."

S T I G M A

57   "only part of the story": Philip Alcabes, "The Ordinariness
       of AIDS," *American Scholar*, Summer 2006, 18–32, http://
       theamericanscholar.org/the-ordinariness-of-aids.

65   "undesired differentness": Erving Goffman, *Stigma: Notes
       on the Management of Spoiled Identity* (New York: Simon &
       Schuster, 1986), p. 4.

68   "Dearly beloved": Michel Foucault, *The History of Madness*,
       trans. Jean Khalfa (London: Routledge, 2006), p. 63.

69   "dominant religious discourse": Daniel Jordan Smith, "Youth,
       Sin and Sex in Nigeria: Christianity and HIV/AIDS-Related
       Beliefs and Behaviour among Rural-Urban Migrants," *Cul-
       ture, Health & Sexuality* 6 (2004), no. 5: 425–37 (p. 430).

69   "sinful immoral lives": Ibid., 429.

71   "AIDS is God's way of checking": Ibid., 430.

72   "Black shapes crouched": Joseph Conrad, *Heart of Darkness*
       and *The Secret Sharer* (New York: Signet Classics, 1997), 83.

73   "continent of AIDS orphans": Christiane Amanpour, CNN
       Presents, *Where Have All the Parents Gone?* CNN, Sep-
       tember 23, 2006, excerpt, YouTube, www.youtube.com
       /watch?v=zdDIZW0WkKA.

75   "Traditional Ways Spread AIDS": Elisabeth Rosenthal, "Traditional Ways Spread AIDS in Africa, Experts Say," *New York Times*, Nov. 21, 2006, www.nytimes.com/2006/11/21 /world/africa/21cameroon.html?pagewanted=all.

76   move between populations: Michael Specter, "The Doomsday Strain," *New Yorker*, Dec. 20, 2010, pp. 50–63, www .gvfi.org/docs/Specter%2012-20-10.pdf.

76   "endemicity of disease": Paul Farmer, *AIDS and Accusation: Haiti and the Geography of Blame* (Berkeley: University of California Press, 2006), 222.

78   "the stage of social impact": Elizabeth Fee and Manon Parry, "Jonathan Mann, HIV/AIDS, and Human Rights," *Journal of Public Health Policy* 29 (2008): 54–71.

SEX

94   35.6 percent of sex workers: *National HIV/AIDS & Reproductive Health Survey*, Federal Ministry of Health, Abuja, 2006.

94   "not only of sexual excess": Susan Sontag, *Illness as Metaphor and AIDS and Its Metaphors* (New York: Picador, 1989), 114.

95   "*this* disease's version of 'the general population'": Ibid., 115.

95   "gay plague": David Black, *The Plague Years: A Chronicle of AIDS, the Epidemic of Our Times* (New York: Simon & Schuster, 1986).

96   African sexuality as Other: Marc Epprecht, *Heterosexual Africa? The History of an Idea from the Age of Exploration to the Age of AIDS* (Athens: Ohio University Press, 2008).

97   "promiscuous by Western standards": Daniel B. Hrdy, "Cultural Practices Contributing to the Transmission of Human Immunodeficiency Virus in Africa," *Reviews of Infectious Diseases* 9, no. 6 (Nov.–Dec. 1987): 1109–19.

98   "not found in the Eurasian system": John C. Caldwell, Pat Caldwell, and Pat Quiggin, "The Social Context of AIDS in Sub-Saharan Africa," *Population and Development Review* 15 (1989), no. 2: 185–234.

99   "greatest struggle": Anonymous, *Marita; or, The Folly of Love*, ed. Stephanie Newell (Leiden: Koninklike Brill, 2002).

110   sequentially monogamous relationships: Martina Morris and Mirjam Kretzschmar, "Concurrent Partnerships and the Spread of HIV," *AIDS* 11 (1997): 641–48.

110   concurrent partnerships: Adaora A. Adimora and Victor J. Schoenbach, "Contextual Factors and the Black-White Disparity in Heterosexual HIV Transmission," *Epidemiology* 13 (2002), no. 6: 707–12.

110   "the speed with which the epidemic spreads": Morris and Kretzschmar, "Concurrent Partnerships."

112   multiple or concurrent partnerships: *National HIV/AIDS & Reproductive Health Survey.*

113   rises to 77 percent: A. O. Arowojulu, A. O. Ilesanmi, O. A. Roberts, and M. A. Okunola, "Sexuality, Contraceptive Choice and AIDS Awareness among Nigerian Undergraduates," *African Journal of Reproductive Health* 6 (2002), no. 2: 60–70.

115   "'shared pleasure' has gained prominence": Eleanor Maticka-Tyndale, Richmond Tiemoko, and Paulina Makinwa-Adebusoye, eds., *Human Sexuality in Africa: Beyond Reproduction* (Auckland Park, South Africa: Fanele/Jacana Media, 2007).

118   900 million condoms: "909.5m Condom Packets Sold in Nigeria," *Nigeria Daily News*, Jan. 31, 2008, http://ndn.nigeria dailynews.com/templates/?a=5879.

124   moral partnering: Daniel Jordan Smith, "Youth, Sin and Sex in Nigeria: Christianity and HIV/AIDS-Related Beliefs and Behaviour among Rural-Urban Migrants," *Culture, Health & Sexuality* 6 (2004), no. 5: 425–37.

126   positive moral connotations: Ibid., 431.

126   more than one moral partner: Ibid., 432.

127   Condom usage is not high: Ibid., 431.

DEATH

139   1.3 million people: *AIDS Epidemic Update 09* (Geneva: Joint United Nations Programme on HIV/AIDS, Nov. 2009), http://data.unaids.org/pub/report/2009/jc1700_epi_up date_2009_en.pdf; *UNAIDS World AIDS Day Report 2011* (Geneva: Joint United Nations Programme on HIV/AIDS, 2011), www.unaids.org/en/media/unaids/contentassets/docu ments/unaidspublication/2011/JC2216_WorldAIDSday_re port_2011_en.pdf; *National Policy on HIV/AIDS*, Federal Government of Nigeria, 2009, http://nigeria.unfpa.org/pdf/ntpol .pdf.

139   two hundred thousand AIDS-related deaths: *AIDS Epidemic Update 09*; *National Policy on HIV/AIDS*.

140   among the sexually active: Markus Haacker, ed., *The Macro-economics of HIV/AIDS* (Washington, DC: International Monetary Fund, 2004), 2.

140   more vulnerable to HIV: Ibid., 23.

140   astoundingly brief forty-five years: *National HIV/AIDS & Reproductive Health Survey*, Federal Ministry of Health, Abuja, 2006.

141   declining workforce: Haacker, *Macroeconomics of HIV/AIDS*, 37.

141   Household incomes drop dramatically: Ibid., 47.

145   ceremony and ritual: Georges Bataille, *Erotism: Death and Sensuality* (San Francisco: City Lights Books, 1986), 44.

150   "Claiming positive identity": Jean Comaroff, "Beyond the Politics of Bare Life: AIDS, (Bio)Politics, and the Neoliberal Order," *Public Culture* 19 (2007), no. 1: 197–221.

SPEAKING OF AIDS

155   "the Nigerian invented noise": Peter Enahoro, *How to Be a Nigerian* (Ibadan, Nigeria: Spectrum Books and Safari Books, 1998).

157   "safe-sex educator's nightmare": Mark Schoofs, "A Tale of
       Two Brothers," part 2, *Village Voice*, Nov. 9, 1999, www
       .villagevoice.com/1999-11-09/news/part-2-a-tale-of-two
       -brothers/3.

HEALING

191   dropped by 20 percent: *UNAIDS Report on the Global AIDS
       Epidemic* (Geneva: Joint United Nations Programme on
       HIV/AIDS, 2010).

191   decreased by about 20 percent: Ibid.

191   the numbers are not rising: Ibid.

193   ten thousand dollars: Kelly A. Gebo, John A. Fleishman,
       Richard Conviser, James Hellinger, Fred J. Hellinger, Joshua
       S. Josephs, Philip Keiser, Paul Gaist, and Richard D. Moore,
       "Contemporary Costs of HIV Healthcare in the HAART
       Era," *AIDS* 24 (2010), no. 17: 2705–15.

197   "creation of a Global AIDS Fund": Abuja Declaration on
       HIV/AIDS, Tuberculosis and Other Related Infectious
       Diseases, Apr. 27, 2001, http://wwwupdate.un.org/ga/aids
       /pdf/abuja_declaration.pdf.

207   "a shared sense of humanity": Lawrence Blum, "Compas-
       sion," in *Explaining Emotions*, ed. Amélie Oksenberg Rorty
       (Berkeley: University of California Press, 1980) 507-18